BEYOND
BOTOX

BEYOND BOTOX

7 STRATEGIES FOR SEXY, AGELESS SKIN
WITHOUT NEEDLES OR SURGERY

BEN AND HOWARD KAMINSKY

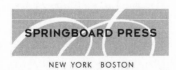

SPRINGBOARD PRESS

NEW YORK BOSTON

We dedicate this book to the thousands of women who have called and written us with real and often anguished questions regarding their skin care needs. We hope this book will help them and all women make more informed choices to take better care of their skin.

Springboard Press

Hachette Book Group USA
1271 Avenue of the Americas, New York, NY 10020

Visit our Web site at www.HachetteBookGroupUSA.com

Springboard Press is an imprint of Warner Books, Inc. The Springboard name and logo are trademarks of Hachette Book Group USA.

First Edition: October 2006

BOTOX® is a registered trademark of Allergan Inc. and is not affiliated in any way with B. Kamins, Chemist, or Hachette Book Group USA.

Library of Congress Cataloging-in-Publication Data
Kaminsky, Ben.
    Beyond Botox : 7 strategies for sexy, ageless skin without needles or surgery / Ben and Howard Kaminsky.
        p.   cm.
    Includes bibliographical references and index.
    ISBN-13: 978-0-8212-8002-7
    ISBN-10: 0-8212-8002-3
    1. Skin — Care and hygiene.   I. Kaminsky, Howard.   II. Title.
RL87.K26   2006
646.7'2 — dc22   2006009388

Q-FF

Printed in the United States of America

Contents

PART I:

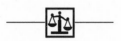

Skin 101

Before you embark on a skin care game plan, it is imperative that you understand all about your skin — the body's largest and most visible organ. In Part I, we will give the background information, definitions, and educational tools necessary to implement the Beyond Botox program in Part II.

Chapter 1

What's Wrong with Botox?

Everything They Don't Want You to Know . . . and Only a Chemist Will Tell You

You look in the mirror on Monday morning and see the face of a middle-aged woman peering back at you. Who is that tired-looking person? Sure, you're not as young as you used to be . . . and the small "laugh lines" around your mouth and eyes don't really bother you too much. They're the signs of a life well lived, right?

But it's your complexion — which always seems dull these days — and those persistent, deeper creases on your forehead that really get you down and make you feel, well, *old*. Maybe your physician is right. Maybe it's time to look into Botox. But ugh, the idea of injecting a toxin like botulism into your face seems downright foolish. Doesn't Joan in the office know someone who had some awful side effects from that procedure?

Sighing, you hop into the shower, hurriedly dress, grab a bagel and a coffee on the way to the office, and spend the day trying to keep up with the crazy rat race that is your life. At night, despite your best intentions, you forgo the gym to stay late at the office, then you rush home for some takeout with the family before crashing into bed . . . and getting up early the next morning to do it all again.

*   *   *

What if I told you that you didn't have to subject yourself to procedures like Botox, Restalin, brow lifts, or other invasive or surgical procedures to have sexy, vibrant, young-looking skin? What if I told you that some doctors — despite their good intentions — actually make big bucks off these types of cosmetic procedures even though there are other, affordable techniques that are even safer and more responsible in the long term? What if I showed you another way to make your skin look beautiful and ageless?

My name is Ben Kaminsky. I am a pharmaceutical and dermatological chemist, cofounder of the cosmeceutical company B. Kamins, Chemist, and president of Odan Laboratories. For more than thirty years, I have been in my laboratory, developing medicines and dermatological preparations that are prescribed by physicians and widely used in hospitals to treat skin conditions and other medical problems. I also formulate very specific *cosmeceuticals*, the cosmetic products that have healing druglike benefits and are intended as a bridge between the physician's office and traditional cosmetics. My chemist colleagues and I are on the front lines of skin care research: we test new products, develop new formulations, and relay that information to your doctor so he or she can learn about the newest advances in beauty, cosmeceuticals, and skin care.

Although dermatologists and other physicians diagnose skin conditions, most doctors have varying knowledge in how to actually treat skin problems, depending on the courses they took in medical school. In fact, it is the pharmaceutical chemist — *the professional who researches and develops the precise formulations* — who ultimately understands how to resolve skin disorders safely and effectively and who helps dermatologists and other medical doctors do the same. That's the work that I do every single day, and I'm thrilled to have the chance to bring my findings directly to the consumer — to you — and let you know the truth about what products, procedures, and lifestyle choices *really* make the most difference for your skin.

The Truth About Botox

Since I started my pharmaceutical career in the early 1970s, we have learned much about skin care and what ingredients are most effective. I have seen tremendous advances in moisturizing materials and in methods to renew aging skin, and we are constantly improving our older formulations to produce revolutionary new products that are far more effective in rejuvenating aging skin and healing dermatological problems than ever before. In particular, we've discovered several topical formulations (i.e., products that can be applied directly to the skin) that are remarkably effective in combating the signs of aging. In addition, certain lifestyle changes (like eating specific foods and maintaining a proper sleep regimen) have dramatic and lasting effects on the skin.

But even as we learn more about what really works to keep skin looking healthy and gorgeous, I have observed an ever-increasing tendency for many physicians and cosmetic dermatologists to turn away from such topical formulations and lifestyle recommendations. Instead, many medical doctors lean toward invasive procedures to rejuvenate aging skin, such as the currently trendy injections of Botox. Botox, as you surely know by now, is a highly diluted and purified form of botulinum toxin (a neurotoxin that causes botulism). When injected into the skin, Botox temporarily reduces the ability of the underlying muscles to contract and crease the skin.

These days, it's hard to open a magazine or turn on the television without seeing an advertisement for Botox or hearing about a glamorous Hollywood star who has reportedly used the procedure. Because of a multimillion-dollar marketing campaign, the money to be made from providing Botox, and, yes, the procedure's sometimes dramatic short-term effects, we are left with the impression that Botox is the cure-all for revitalizing aging skin.

The results, admittedly, can be dramatic . . . in the short term. In the past five years, the use of Botox has caught the imagination of numerous physicians who now offer it to their patients, both young and old, as a "quick fix" wrinkle treatment. However, I strongly believe that not everyone is a candidate for such an invasive procedure, and I respectfully but firmly disagree with those doctors who tout Botox as the only effective long-term solution. The effects of Botox are temporary — and in some cases even harmful — and this type of quick fix is not the secret to long-lasting, beautiful skin. I believe that there's a safer and ultimately more effective alternative.

What goes underreported about Botox is the fact that, as with all relatively new procedures, there are certain risks involved. Many times these Botox injections can even cause unwanted side effects. For instance, some patients have the tendency to bleed and bruise easily. They also may be slow to heal, allergic to the injected ingredients, or have difficulty with the topical anesthetics. Although it happens rarely, there is a risk that the doctor slips a bit when injecting Botox — and the consequences of this can be dire. The worst that can happen is that you won't be able to raise your eyelids all the way, or, if the shot was near the mouth (which is unapproved usage according to the FDA), you could be left drooling. If this occurs, you would have to wait for the toxin to wear off, which can take several months. Moreover, because the toxin actually paralyzes the muscles that cause deep frown lines, even if the doctor did a perfect job, you might not be able to frown, raise your eyebrows, or squint. This could lead to a diminished range of facial expressions, so you might want to consider that too.

And if your wrinkles and/or sagging skin are resulting from loss of elasticity that occurs with aging, sun exposure, and smoking, sometimes Botox won't work at all. There are other treatments for such conditions. Just keep in mind that Botox isn't a miraculous cure for all wrinkles.

In addition to checking to make sure you're not allergic to any of the ingredients in Botox Cosmetic, you should not use Botox if you have an infection where you want it injected, or if you are pregnant or think you might be pregnant. Also discuss with your doctor any medications you're taking. And though the Food and Drug Administration (FDA) has approved Botox Cosmetic to temporarily improve the appearance of moderate to severe frown lines between the eyebrows (called glabellar lines), the FDA also warns that "the most common adverse events following injection are headache, respiratory infection, flu syndrome, blepharoptosis (droopy eyelids), and nausea. Less frequent adverse reactions (less than 3 percent of patients) included pain in the face, redness at the injection site, and muscle weakness. These reactions were generally temporary, but could last several months. Because Botox Cosmetic is a prescription drug, it must be used carefully under medical supervision." For a supposedly "safe" elective procedure, this is scary stuff!

Despite all the press and hype, only 2 percent of women in the United States used Botox last year. The other 98 percent went "beyond Botox," instead opting for noninvasive topical treatments and healing lifestyle therapies to resolve problematic or aging skin.

The bottom line is this: Botox is *not* the cure-all for sun-damaged skin or the wrinkles associated with aging; there are other alternatives.

Miracle Cures or Marketing Myths?

The FDA cautions that the recent rise in the popularity of Botox has much to do with the manner in which it is marketed. For instance, some practitioners buy the toxin in bulk and arrange get-togethers (called Botox parties) for people who want to receive treatments. As in business, volume discounts are available in medicine. Not only has the FDA voiced great concern that Botox has the potential for misuse and abuse, the American Society for Aesthetic Plastic Surgery (ASAPS) recently reported that unqualified people are dispensing Botox in salons, gyms, hotel rooms, home-based offices, and other retail venues. In such cases, consumers run the risk of improper technique, inappropriate dosage, and unsanitary conditions.

Maintaining the smooth "Botoxed" face is also an expensive proposition. Most print and television ads do *not* tell consumers that to maintain the anti-wrinkle effect, Botox shots are necessary approximately every three to four months, costing from $350 to $500 for a single injection, $400 to $900 for areas requiring more than one injection, and $600 to $1,300 for larger surfaces such as forehead wrinkles. On an added note, contrary to what some experts claim, there are now those who advise that Botox injections may result in the development of new wrinkles as nearby muscles "over-compensate," creating new facial expressions in the area where the muscles are paralyzed.

For dermatological purposes, Botox is only approved by the FDA to reduce the severity of frown lines (for up to 120 days). Yet hundreds of dermatology and medical Web sites found on Google widely advertise the use of Botox for treating myriad cosmetic conditions such as brow furrow, crow's-feet, forehead creases, and neck bands. When the botulinum toxin was improperly used, there have been cases of paralysis and even deaths after an injection. You might remember the widely publicized story in late 2004 about the Palm Beach County, Florida, osteopath, his girlfriend, and another couple who were paralyzed and put on ventilators after being injected with a "cheap alternative to Botox." It was revealed that the ill people had contracted botulism, a rare disease that is fatal in 10 percent of cases. In another case in 2003, a Florida woman went into cardiac arrest after receiving a Botox injection, dying shortly thereafter. The cause of death was listed as anaphylactic shock associated with Botox injection.

Don't get me wrong. Along with Botox injections and cosmetic procedures, many physicians prescribe numerous topical therapies. We all know the big names in this skin care field — celebrity dermatologists with pricey products and quick-fix plans to make you look younger yesterday. Some of them have good things to say and good products to promote. In fact, not a week goes by that I don't get a call from a dermatologist or his or her agent asking me if I would be interested in formulating a line of topical skin-treatment products for use under the physician's name. When I ask the good doctor if he or she wants to build upon his or her clinical studies or revolutionary findings acquired in years of medical practice, the answer is usually no. It then becomes apparent that these medical doctors realize that there is a significant financial benefit to combining business and medicine, and they are looking for a way to get into the retail skin game. My response to them is always "Thank you for thinking of me, but no, thanks."

The reality of skin care today is that many of these self-promoting physicians are successful as both marketing executives *and* doctors. Their use of the media is brilliant; it is easy to use ostentatious terminology when addressing a captive nonprofessional audience. The talk is impressive, the promises are grandiose, and people think that the flamboyant health care professionals surely know what they are talking about . . . or do they?

One such popular dermatologist turned entrepreneur and anti-aging author has extensively touted the use of alpha lipoic acid as "a quintessential antioxidant, anti-aging ingredient." Yet new findings on alpha lipoic acid by Dr. Jing-Yi Lin with the Department of Dermatology at Chang Gung Memorial Hospital in Taipei, Taiwan, contradict these claims. In extensive research published in the November 2004 issue of the *Journal of Investigative Dermatology*, Dr. Lin concludes that this nutrient is completely ineffective as a topical antioxidant, contradicting the previous "hyped" benefits of alpha lipoic. The aforementioned anti-aging author also recommends megadoses (400 to 800 International Units [IU] daily) of vitamin E in all of his anti-aging books, when in fact this is contrary to the latest scientific findings. Reports from the American Heart Association at their Scientific Sessions in 2004 state that high doses of vitamin E supplements "do more harm than good, can *increase the risk of death*, and should be avoided." By the way, the American Heart Association defines a high dose as over 400 IUs daily (the lowest starting dose in the doctor's prescriptive program).

So where does the truth lie? How can a consumer know what is truth and what is marketing hype? Many marketing-savvy executives use cosmetics studies to hype claims for anti-aging skin products, promoting them as magic potions for young-looking skin. The fact is, many of these cosmetics studies do not mimic the hard scientific work required for approval by the FDA, and the result is a shelf full of cosmeceutical products that are of questionable value to you, the consumer.

Confidence in a Chemist's Perspective

I am not a dermatologist. For more than three decades, I've worked as a pharmaceutical chemist — on the front lines of the skin care industry, making and testing and perfecting the products that your dermatologist prescribes. During this time, I have become increasingly distressed to see the hype that many cosmetic dermatologists and skin care companies use in advertisements simply to sell products. And the products they sell are not cheap. In the United States alone, more than $45 billion is spent annually on cosmetics and toiletries. This amount does not include the billions spent on doctor-prescribed therapies for the skin. With highly scientific words such as *retinoids, hyaluronic acid, nonosomes,* and *liposomes* appearing in product ingredient lists, is it any wonder that most women are confused and even overwhelmed when it comes to making responsible choices for their skin?

From the time I started my pharmaceutical company, I have observed specialists touting many topical products they claim to have formulated but which they have actually purchased from private-label contractors — not pharmaceutical labs. Consumers do not realize that many of these dermatologists and other physicians who claim to have found the "magical treatment" for aging skin are actually selling the exact same topical product as their counterparts but with their own brand names stamped on the packaging! The problem arises because dermatologists and physicians are specifically trained in medical school as *diagnosticians* — professionals who identify skin conditions such as aging or wrinkling skin, sun-damaged skin, acne, eczema, rosacea, and skin cancers — and *not* as *chemists* — scientists who understand the composition, structure, and properties of substances and the transformations they undergo when formulated into medications and dermatological treatments.

Many in the health care profession believe there is a potential conflict of interest when cosmetic dermatologists practice medicine along with selling their own brand of topical "formulations." I firmly believe, as do many clinical dermatologists, that these doctors compromise their reputation as medical professionals when they add marketing their cosmetic wares to the practice of medicine. When I see doctors marketing their topical products, it also leads me to the disturbing conclusion that much of the popularity of topical products has to do with the marketing rather than the therapeutic formulation.

Devising a cosmeceutical to alleviate acne, reduce scars, diminish under-eye puffiness, or reverse the obvious signs of aging is both an art and a science. The chemist fully understands atoms and molecules and how matter interacts with matter in the classic chemical reaction. The pharmaceutical chemist comprehends how chemical substances interact with living systems and which compounds have medicinal value, including the composition, properties, interactions, toxicology, and desirable effects.

Once the chemist has researched and developed a new product over a period of years, the pharmaceutical companies further study this compound in clinical trials before marketing it to doctors, who then prescribe the product for consumers (patients). During every stage of scientific research and development, the chemist and pharmaceutical company work side by side to perfect the formulation before marketing it to doctors and consumers, making sure they fully understand how it is used, including the dose, the side effects, and the contraindications, among other factors.

Does everyone in the skin care industry give consumers an honest appraisal of a product's benefits and risks? As a scientist and chemist, I think the answer is no, and this causes me great distress. I remember attending a skin care convention in the late 1990s and being appalled at the faulty or blatantly misleading information leaders in the cosmeceutical industry were giving consumers. They were cleverly deceiving both media and customers, with, I imagine, the intent of profiting from their cosmetics and the skin care products they had formulated. Not only did the exaggerated claims indicate a cynical, irresponsible marketing ploy, but they also made the skin care field appear to be solely a business rather than a medical profession where trained professionals are passionate about the health and well-being of consumers.

Quality Control and My Own Family

In addition to being fervent about my profession, I am devoted to my family and absolutely in love with my wife, children, and grandchildren. Like most of you, I constantly worry about my family's health, particularly their skin problems. I want to make sure my children and grandchildren are using products without harsh ingredients that can wreak havoc on delicate skin and with adequate protection against the sun's ultraviolet (UV) rays.

For years prior to starting the B. Kamins line of cosmeceuticals, I had been formulating topical preparations for the needs of my young family. I started with diaper rash ointments when our children were newborns and moved into personalized poison ivy lotions, shampoos, hair conditioners, and even fragrance-free body lotions for my wife and daughter. I formulated outstanding and gentle acne gels for my teenagers that did not leave their skin inflamed as the popular gels did, and I prepared a variety of sunscreens for my kids' sensitive skin.

But for my family — as well as in my professional career — I am extremely conservative about recommending treatment unless there is scientific proof that it is necessary. As an example, our first child, Howard, was a fair-skinned, hazel-eyed, redheaded baby. As a young, inexperienced parent in the early 1960s, my lovely wife, Mildred, kept Howard sleeping in the sun for a period of time each day, which resulted in unintended skin reddening. My wife's phone call to our competent, friendly pediatrician resulted in a scolding and a prescription for a sunscreening lotion containing para-aminobenzoic acid (PABA). Quite distraught, Mildred immediately called me at the lab to tell me about the scolding. She also mentioned the prescription for a PABA sunscreen, which was being used extensively in North America at the time.

In my lab, I had myself been working on topical preparations to protect the skin from heightened sensitivity to the sun's ultraviolet radiation for patients who were taking various categories of medications including antidepressants, tranquilizers, diabetic medications, anticonception drugs, and antibiotics. After reviewing some adverse clinical findings regarding PABA, I had chosen not to include this ingredient in my own sunscreen formulations. I remember telling Mildred to hold off filling the PABA sunscreen prescription.

That evening, I brought home a preparation I had been working on in the lab. My sunscreen preparation contained a safe formulation of titanium dioxide and an octyl salicylate complex. Both these ingredients had been proven safe, nonirritating, and effective sunscreens when used in well-formulated preparations. At that time, few chemists were testing the sun protection factor (SPF) in topical sunscreens, but I believed that the SPF in my preparation was approximately 15, which gives a few (two to three) hours of protection against ultraviolet sun rays.

Later that evening, I called our pediatrician and questioned the use of PABA preparations. I received a standard answer from our kind doctor — that the medical review boards had approved the product, and who was he (or I, for that matter!) to question their wisdom. Despite his advice, we didn't use the PABA-based sunscreen and instead used my formulation. I learned early on in my career as a pharmaceutical chemist that it takes time and sometimes repeated bad experiences for doctors' prescribing habits to change. Often, topical therapies worsen skin conditions until there are enough complaints and the review boards halt the product and call for change. Today we know that PABA causes both sensory and visual skin problems, including rashes, itching, tingling, and redness. Nowadays, sunscreens do not usually contain this ingredient.

The point is this: even though we call on our medical doctors seeking treatment for symptoms, and despite their best intentions, they don't always get it right. What they do know is that patients expect something from them; they are often hard-pressed to prescribe medications, which is why antibiotics, procedures, and products are often overprescribed and misused.

A Cosmeceutical and Lifestyle Approach

Over the years, as I created more and more cosmeceuticals for our family's needs and even therapies for friends and colleagues, I began to realize that these topical treatments could offer tremendous benefit to others too. In 1997, my son Howard and I cofounded B. Kamins, Chemist, an innovative skin care collection and a pioneer in the cosmeceutical industry. Howard has a business degree from McGill University, a law degree (LLB) from the University of Sherbrooke (Canada), and an LLM from Notre Dame Law School (Indiana). Apart from being an attorney turned entrepreneur–marketing executive, Howard is a very devoted husband to Laurie and father of three-year-old Isabelle (and a new one on the way).

While I toiled in the lab, Howard made it his goal to build the B. Kamins brand with a personal touch. He went door-to-door to spas and specialty stores throughout the Northeast and educated anyone who would listen about responsible skin care. Today, as CEO of B. Kamins, Chemist, Howard manages the multimillion-dollar corporation from our offices in New York City and spends what little downtime he has with his family.

Whether lecturing to professional societies or cosmeceutical and skin care organizations, or talking with the personnel at day spas, medical spas, or resort spas, Howard and I continually remind professionals and consumers that there is no one-size-fits-all approach when it comes to dealing sensibly with skin care problems. What might work to resolve your colleague's skin problem may cause a rash or sudden outbreak of pimples on your skin.

No matter how much you hydrate or exfoliate, skin does age — and sometimes well before its time. That's why we promote a combined cosmeceutical and lifestyle approach to having sexy, ageless skin. No doubt, the sun caused most of the skin damage you see on your skin right now. But smoking cigarettes, drinking too much alcohol, extreme temperatures, and a host of noxious chemicals and pollutants in the air outside can also damage skin. Chronic stress is another known skin irritant that can make your skin highly reactive and result in outbreaks of pimples, acne, or rosacea at most inappropriate times. Lack of sleep makes your skin puffy, ashen, and pale, and accentuates the deep reddish blue of under-eye circles. A poor diet lacking in immune-boosting nutrients can make your skin appear sallow, overly dry, or even too oily. And exercise obsession can result in hormone imbalance even in college-age women, which can lead to osteopenia (pre-osteoporosis), with thin bones that fracture easily. Strong bones are essential to stretch your skin and keep it taut through the years, and tight skin is younger-looking skin.

So where do you begin? A reasonable approach to understanding and treating skin in each stage of the life cycle is critical. And finding that proper balance — a responsible, noninvasive program that you can adapt to your unique skin care problems and that also empowers you to play an active role in improving and protecting your health — is the purpose of *Beyond Botox*.

How *Beyond Botox* Can Help You Right Now

Unlike other books on aging skin, this book places you, the reader, center stage by focusing on where you are in your life cycle and identifying your risks for particular skin problems. For example, pregnant women can have darkened pigmentation on the face and bright red spider veins, while women in the perimenopause years (the two to eight years preceding menopause) may have the beginnings of fine lines and wrinkles and under-eye bags. Women in menopause (around age fifty-one) contend with blotchy, thinning, and transparent skin, as well as added dryness, flaking, and dark age spots on the face, arms, and hands. Still, no matter what your life stage or skin problem, there are *noninvasive* answers in this book.

As you read the book, you will see that it quickly moves beyond a discussion of skin basics and how I formulate cosmeceuticals in my Montreal-based lab to page after page of skin-saving strategies that you can use right now to have sexy, ageless skin.

In chapter 2, "What's Your Skin's Real Age?," we discuss the skin and how it represents a unique "fingerprint" of what goes on inside (and outside) your body. We will explain what occurs when skin ages and what you can do to stop it. You'll learn how specific risk factors (such as sun exposure and even the way you sleep at night) predispose you to visible signs of premature skin aging. And at the end of the chapter, you'll take a "Real Skin Age Quiz" to find out your skin's true age and determine which risk factors you can change *right now* to slow or even reverse your skin's aging.

Chapter 3, "What's in Your Medicine Cabinet?," is a most crucial chapter. I'll take you into my lab and introduce you to my passion: understanding how to best treat women's skin. I believe that cosmeceuticals, when properly formulated and properly used, are the future of skin care. Here I will help you appraise the various ingredients used in your own creams and lotions and let you know if a product has merit or is nothing but marketing hype. You'll learn how to go to the drugstore or cosmetics counter and shop for the perfect products that will complement your skin type and lifestyle . . . and you'll also discover what ingredients to avoid at any cost. After all, why pay money for a product that has no curative value — or may even damage your skin — just because it comes wrapped in a shiny package with a celebrity endorsement? I'll tell you what I tell my children: *always know what you are applying to your skin!*

In Part II, "The Beyond Botox 7-Step Program," Howard and I will explain our renowned, scientifically based lifestyle program, which will help you meet your individual skin care needs with the following strategies:

1. **Nourish:** *Feed your skin from the inside out*
2. **Move:** *Exercise regularly but don't go for the burn*
3. **Rest:** *Get quality sleep to rejuvenate skin*
4. **Relax:** *De-stress to boost skin healing*
5. **Super-Saturate:** *Moisturize properly to quench your skin's thirst*
6. **Pamper:** *Become spa savvy for wellness and balance*
7. **Radiate:** *Combat specific skin problems . . . at any age*

To Sexy, Ageless Skin!

I believe that women today are left in a terribly difficult position — with serious questions about how to handle the myriad skin problems they may face. While women know they will get older, they do not want to look old. Yet without a responsible skin care game plan, including a full understanding of invasive procedures such as Botox, women are putting their skin health in jeopardy and may have to live with less than acceptable results the rest of their lives.

Throughout this book, I will only suggest products that I believe are safe and effective for you and your family members. In that regard, whether you are in your thirties, forties, fifties, sixties, or beyond, I want to give you responsible, stage-specific guidance to help you assess your skin right now and stop — even reverse — the specific problems that keep you from looking youthful and sexy. I believe that everyone must make a personal and lifelong commitment to be the ultimate guardian of his or her skin, focusing on the skin care regimen that fits his or her life stage, lifestyle habits, and skin problems. To that end, this book will provide you with the information and tools you need to determine a balanced skin care approach that works for you and your family.

Together we can do it. Let's get started!

Ben Kaminsky

Chapter 2

What's Your Skin's Real Age?

Your Worst Skin Care Habits . . . and How You Can Change Them

After spending a lifetime in the blistering Santa Monica sun, Lauren, thirty-six, a professional counselor and part-time yoga instructor, is concerned about the rough skin, fine lines, and crow's-feet that seem to have appeared on her face almost overnight. She wonders if it's too late to start being proactive about her skin and lifestyle habits.

Claudia, twenty-nine, from Houston, has lived with blushing apple cheeks her entire life. Recently diagnosed with rosacea, a chronic skin disease that resembles acne and affects 14 million Americans, this young attorney now has dark red patches, small pimples, and broken blood vessels on her face. She asks what she can do to keep this inflammatory condition from worsening.

Elizabeth, sixty-one, from Indianapolis, wants a product that can reverse her postmenopausal skin changes yet is unsure which compounds are safe — and which ones could cause her highly allergic skin to flare.

Immediately after having Botox injections in the forehead area, Arlene, fifty-two, the owner of a New York City boutique and former model, experienced drooping of the upper eyelid (called "partial ptosis"). Though this condition went away after several months, she is now seeking an injection-free topical preparation that targets wrinkles and expression lines and helps to reverse the visible signs of aging associated with menopause.

These are just a few of the thousands of women who have written to me over the past year for immediate answers to problematic and aging skin . . . and they are not alone. With the enormous popularity of beauty-related television programs and every type of extreme makeover imaginable, America has experienced a recent surge in the demand for rejuvenation, as women vow to take control over their lives — and skin aging. Today's "body business" is big business — a massive $40 billion global industry, to be precise.

It must seem surprising that aging skin is even a concern in the twenty-first century. After all, we are a technically sophisticated society with tremendous health advances that have improved the quality and length of our lives. Women get annual preventative mammograms to detect early signs of cancer and begin treatment even before symptoms of the disease are experienced. We now have access to complete joint replacements, cures for once-terminal diseases, and organ transplants that have greatly increased the quality of life and life span for millions. The average American female born in 1900 had a life expectancy of 47 years, and a female born in 1950 was given the life expectancy of 71.1 years. Today, a baby girl has a life expectancy of 84.7 years!

Yet while modern medical innovations are allowing us to live longer lives than ever before, we not only want to live long, we want to live *well*. And part of living well these days involves looking as good on the outside as we feel on the inside. After all, who doesn't want to turn back the hands of time when it comes to our appearance — particularly the appearance of our skin? As one woman said to Howard at a recent cosmeceutical conference: "I am trim, teach a Spinning class at the Y, and own my own company. Even though I am forty-five, I feel like I am twenty years younger. I want my skin to look as young as I feel."

"To look as young as we feel" is the chorus of millions, particularly baby boomers who are used to getting all they can out of life. However, the reality is that even with modern scientific breakthroughs, aging is an inevitable process. And though we may want skin that looks younger, many of us have taken our skin for granted for decades and are just now waking up to the certainty that our skin will age. When you were young, did you ever consider the injurious effect that exposure to the sun's ultraviolet rays might have on your skin? We now realize that more than *80 percent* of the visible signs of aging — the tiny lines around the eyes, blotchy skin tone, brown age spots, and wrinkles — are direct results of the UV rays we were exposed to before the age of eighteen. When you add years of photoaging during the teens, twenties, and thirties to exposure to environmental toxins and pollutants, carcinogens, and extreme temperatures, is it any wonder that premature skin aging is so common among young and middle-aged women in our society?

It's a frustrating situation, but I'm here today with good news for you. While no one can reverse all the damage to skin after decades of abuse, I believe that every woman can look younger than her chronological age — without using Botox or other invasive procedures. You can do this by making specific choices about how you treat or pamper yourself — and your skin — each day. The resulting healthy glow in your face, combined with the increased oomph and vitality you feel, will radiate youthful allure . . . and this *I promise!*

Facing Up to Aging Skin

A quick glance in a mirror is every woman's reality check as she comes face-to-face with skin aging. And the simple truth is this: all the anti-aging creams, exfoliations, Botox injections, and cosmetic procedures will not completely stop the skin changes that occur over time. Even if you *never* exposed your skin to the sun's rays, with aging there is still a loss of fat and breakdown of collagen, the group of proteins found in skin, bones, and other connective tissue, that ultimately results in wrinkles and sagging, transparent skin. That's because your skin, the largest organ in the human body, is an integral part of the immune, nervous, and endocrine systems, and the fingerprint of what is going on *inside* your body.

Consider a newborn's skin. At birth, the infant's skin is soft, lush, and pliable. Over time, the skin firms and thickens. The skin's texture, temperature, color, and clarity all give a wealth of information about your age and current physical condition, keeping no secrets about lifestyle habits, your personal hygiene, whether you smoke or drink, how much time you have spent in the sun, your nutritional and sleep status, and your overall health — *good or bad.*

Through the years, the skin is exposed to damaging ultraviolet rays, chemicals, and extreme temperatures, as well as cellular demise from free radicals. Free radicals are the unstable by-products of oxidation, the chemical process that causes iron to rust and a peeled apple or banana to turn brown. Free radicals can cause similar deterioration in the skin and body, as they destroy cell membranes or make cells vulnerable to decay and pathogens. These free radicals damage your DNA and mitochondria, the basic building blocks of all tissues, and leave in their path the brown age spots and fine lines and wrinkles we all recognize as the signs of aging.

But there are natural ways to combat this damage and even reverse some significant signs of premature skin aging. For an example, eating certain anti-aging "superfoods" that are high in antioxidants and powerful healing compounds (not just popping vitamins and supplements) appears to neutralize these free radicals and take away their destructive power. Many scientists now believe that antioxidants also reduce the risk of some degenerative diseases associated with aging, including very serious skin cancers, and slow down premature skin aging. (In our program's first step, "Nourish," page 55, we've done the homework for you and will discuss the foods highest in antioxidants and other key nutrients to help combat this free radical damage.)

Another way to slow the effects of time on the skin and even reverse some skin damage is to use the proper ingredients on your skin — carefully selecting healing compounds in your lotions, creams, and ointments that fit your skin's needs. For instance, if your skin is ultradry and flaky, we will teach you how to identify the ingredients that are best suited for dry, scaly skin. Or, if you have excessively oily skin that is prone to pimples or acne, finding a topical lotion that moisturizes without being overly greasy can keep your skin healthy without exacerbating your blemishes. We'll learn more about choosing the proper topical treatments for your particular skin in the next chapter.

In this chapter, we'll start by giving you a bit of background information about how healthy skin works and how aging naturally happens to skin. Then I'll offer you a quiz — a simple assessment to see how your chronological age compares to your "skin age." It's a predictor of how healthy your skin is today and how healthy it will be tomorrow, and a guideline for what you should be doing to slow or even reverse the many signs of aging.

Understanding Your Skin

First, just a few words about your skin and how it works. As the body's outer covering, the skin protects the internal organs from heat, light, injury, and infection. It is sensitive to many different kinds of stimuli, such as pain, pressure, temperature, and joint and muscle position. Not only does the skin regulate your body temperature, but it stores water, fat, and vitamin D (a must for keeping your bones and teeth strong).

The skin is composed of three layers: the epidermis, the dermis, and the subcutaneous (or fat) layer. The epidermis, or outermost layer, shows the visible signs of wear and tear. About 95 percent of the cells in the epidermis function to make new skin cells; the other 5 percent make melanin, which gives skin its color. As we age, these epidermis cells replace themselves more slowly (up to 30 to 50 percent more slowly by age fifty).

The middle layer of skin, or the dermis, contains nerve endings, oil and sweat glands, hair follicles, blood vessels, nerve endings, and protein fibers, collagen and elastin, which are strong and stretchy. This layer of skin has sebaceous (oil) glands that produce sebum, the natural oil that keeps skin lubricated and protected. Changes in the dermis occur naturally with aging. For example, cell numbers decrease, and the dermis becomes thinner and less capable of retaining moisture. When the collagen and elastin lose their flexibility, the skin starts to sag and wrinkle.

The subcutaneous is the innermost layer of skin. This layer is made up mostly of fat and helps the body stay warm and protects it from injury. With aging, there is thinning of the subcutaneous layer in certain areas, particularly the face, the hands, and the shins. As this fat layer thins, the skin on the face loses its plumpness, and wrinkles can become more obvious.

Telomeres and Skin Aging

While you might associate aging with what you see on the surface — the wrinkles, brown age spots, and thin or sagging skin — these changes initially happen on a much smaller cellular level. The epidermis is one of the few regenerative tissues in the body with an enzyme called telomerase, which regulates the growth at the ends of chromosomes (bundles of DNA where genetic information is stored). Telomeres are specialized stretches of DNA that cap the ends of human chromosomes, helping to protect them from damage and degradation, and telomerase are the enzymes in the telomeres.

Scientists now believe that telomeres are critical in aging. Each time a cell divides, its telomeres get a little bit shorter. Eventually, if the telomeres become too short to divide, the cell will die. Age-related diseases and premature-aging syndromes are characterized by short telomeres. Some experts have suggested that preserving the telomeres may protect the chromosomes, giving the cell a longer life and slowing the aging process. In other words, telomeres seem to act as a body's "biological clock," stopping cell division and activating aging.

Zeroing in on the impact of telomerase on aging, scientists from the University of Texas Southwestern Medical Center believe that by keeping cells alive and dividing, it may be possible to control age-related disorders ranging from skin wrinkling to some types of blindness — and perhaps even heart disease and autoimmune diseases like rheumatoid arthritis and multiple sclerosis (MS). These researchers have also discovered that when telomerase is added to the chromosomes of cells, the cells continue to divide and show no signs of aging or dying. One day, this work could lead to breakthrough drugs that will stop cells from dying and preserve the functioning of body parts that normally break down as we age.

So what does this mean for your skin? By making smart lifestyle choices, in addition to smart choices about the products you use on your skin, you can slow the degradation of the telomeres in your body and in effect slow down your body's biological clock. It's a pretty exciting promise! But before we examine that further, let's take an assessment to see where you and your skin are right now.

What's Your Skin's "Real Age"?

The reality is that skin does age. But what makes me extremely concerned is seeing how so many people (especially women) speed up the process of skin aging by the lifestyle habits they engage in, such as suntanning, starving to be thin, getting little sleep, and smoking cigarettes. These habits damage the structure of the skin, and over time the ongoing deterioration worsens the skin's appearance. Collagen and elastin are lost from the dermis with normal aging, but when you add poor lifestyle habits, the aging process accelerates. The skin becomes thinner and more fragile, and eventually your body has trouble getting enough moisture to the epidermis, causing wrinkles and sagging skin. This may be quite pronounced in some women, particularly if they are underweight, eat few fruits and vegetables, are smokers, and are constantly in the sun. Over time, the fat in the subcutaneous layer that gives younger skin its plump appearance also begins to disappear, causing the epidermis to sag, and fine lines and deep wrinkles to form. When you add years of unhealthy lifestyle habits to normal skin aging, you can count on looking a lot older than your chronological age.

Skin Age Quiz

Take the Skin Age Quiz to find out how old your skin looks. Check each of the following factors that may trigger premature skin aging. Give yourself 1 point if this describes you and 0 if it does not. Add up your score to determine your skin's age.

1. Mother had premature skin aging
2. Chronic illness such as diabetes or hypothyroidism
3. Osteopenia (early bone loss)
4. Long-term medication use (oral)
5. Normal menopause
6. Surgical menopause before age forty
7. History of poorly treated acne
8. History of poorly treated rosacea
9. Pale, freckled skin
10. Fair skin with tiny pores and/or moles
11. Noticeable fine lines and wrinkles before age thirty-five
12. Obese (more than 10 percent over normal weight)
13. Underweight (ten or more pounds less than normal weight)

(continued)

14. History of dieting deprivation (too few calories)
15. History of binge dieting (losing and gaining the same ten to twenty pounds)
16. Diet high in processed foods with few fruits and vegetables
17. High-fat diet
18. Cigarette smoker
19. Secondhand smoke
20. Heavy alcohol use (more than five or more drinks on the same occasion on each of five or more days in the past thirty days)
21. History of excessive exercise
22. Sedentary lifestyle (little exercise)
23. High-stress lifestyle
24. Personal history of precancerous skin lesions and/or skin cancer
25. Less than six hours of sleep each night
26. History of excessive sun exposure, inability to tan, and sun-induced freckles
27. Blistering sunburns in the first two decades of life
28. Infrequent use of sunscreen during childhood and adult years
29. Use of tanning salons
30. Poor skin care hygiene and infrequent use of moisturizers

Now total up your score:

21–30: Add *ten years* to your real age to get your skin age. Your high score indicates your skin may be paying the price for years of neglect. Take advantage of the information in the seven Beyond Botox strategies (Part II of the book) to change your lifestyle habits and halt or even reverse some outward signs of skin aging.

14–20: Add *six years* to your real age to get your skin age. Although you've led a fairly healthy life, there are some lifestyle habits that still need your focus. Review the suggestions at the end of each strategy, particularly strategies 1 through 4, to see what else you can do to have younger-looking skin.

6–13: Add *three years* to your real age to get your skin age. While there is not a lot of disparity between your skin age and your real

(continued)

age, it doesn't hurt to focus on those healthy behaviors you might have ignored. Do you need to increase fruits and vegetables in your daily diet? Exercise regularly but not excessively? Perhaps you need to reduce stress before it "gets under your skin." Find helpful tips in the seven strategies and use these to your skin's advantage.

0–5: Your skin age is your *real age*. Congratulations! You have aged well, and your skin reflects the healthy lifestyle choices you have made over the past decades. Continue to make excellent choices in how you treat yourself and be sure to take time to pamper yourself and care for those skin problems that are common in women (strategies 6 and 7).

Assessing the Damage to Your Skin

What has caused the skin changes you see? There are two types of factors that affect how your skin will age. Intrinsic aging is caused by the genes you inherit and is pretty much set in stone. This means if your parents aged well, chances are that you will too — especially if you continue to take care of yourself with our Beyond Botox seven-step lifestyle program and use the proper ingredients to moisturize your skin. Extrinsic aging is caused by lifestyle habits and photoaging. We believe that every woman can assess her lifestyle habits and change those over which she has control, especially her exposure to the sun's ultraviolet radiation, which appears to be the most critical and damaging factor.

Intrinsic Aging: Like Mother, Like Daughter

Intrinsic, or genetic, aging begins in the midtwenties, when collagen production slows and elastin, the substance that causes skin to snap back into place, has less snap. Your genetic clock appears to activate this process at a predetermined time — remember those telomeres we talked about earlier? — because these types of changes in the skin typically appear at the same time you start to notice degenerative changes in other body organs. The diminished production of collagen results in fine lines and wrinkles. You might first notice these lines around the eyes (called crow's-feet). Over time, they are evident on the forehead, eyelids, mouth (laugh lines), neck, and jaw.

During this aging process, there is a decrease in the number of immune cells, resulting in a reduced capacity to fight infections. Many women begin to notice tiny blood vessels on the cheeks and nose, as well as increased pigmentation (brown age spots and a blotchy complexion) in sun-exposed areas of the skin. With age and the decline of the skin's immunity, skin tumors (both benign and malignant) become more frequent, as do small growths (skin tags) that are unsightly and can become irritated when rubbed.

Other outward signs of intrinsic aging include loss of underlying fat, thin and transparent skin, dry skin that may itch, and hair loss. As the skin's fat padding decreases, there is an increased chance of bruising and skin tearing, particularly on the arms and hands.

Over time, the collagen and elastin in the connective tissues of the skin weaken and diminish. The skin loses its elasticity and smoothness. Wrinkles that started as tiny lines transform into deep creases in the skin, and the skin along the jowls begins to sag. Initially, wrinkles are more pronounced on areas near the eyes and lips. With increasing age, they become apparent on the neck and ears. It's a sobering picture, and the fact is that if you are lucky enough to live to a ripe old age, this process will happen to you. But it's the *extrinsic* factors — the lifestyle factors that you can control — that will help determine whether these aging symptoms happen earlier or later for you.

Extrinsic Aging: The Factors You Can Control

Extrinsic aging is an entirely separate process and is triggered by years of damage from the sun and wind, smoking, gravity, and more. The *sun alone* is to blame for freckles, age spots, spider veins, leathery skin, loose skin, and actinic keratoses, the thick, rough growths on sun-exposed skin. Pay attention, because this is the vital information, the tips on what you can do to start lessening or even reversing the age your skin appears to be.

Although you have no control over genetics or your age, you can guard your skin against the wrinkles, fine lines, roughness, and other damage caused by extrinsic aging. If your skin is damaged as a result of extrinsic aging, there are very specific lifestyle strategies in our program, along with topical therapies, that can help slow down aging and even reverse some of the damage you see. Let's look at some skin-aging factors over which you have control:

Environmental damage. Exposure to the sun, wind, and other elements causes more than *80 percent* of the damage on the face, resulting in deep lines and wrinkles, thickened skin, discoloration, and even skin cancer. More than 1.3 million new cases of skin cancer are diagnosed in the United States annually. It is estimated that more than 50 percent of Americans will have skin cancer at some point in their lives.

Soft as a Baby's . . .

If you really want to see how environmental damages triggers premature skin aging, compare the skin on your face to that on your buttocks. Because the buttocks are rarely exposed to the sun (at least on most of us!), they show only the effects of intrinsic, or normal, aging. Your face, neck, chest, arms, and hands all show the damage caused by exposure to the environment, particularly the sun's ultraviolet rays. So unless you've done excessive sunbathing in a thong, this is a good benchmark for how your skin *could* look . . . if you take great care of it.

Lifestyle habits. Extrinsic skin aging is linked to lifestyle habits such as deprivation dieting, exercise obsession, excessive alcohol drinking, and sleep deficit. (We address all of these in our program.)

Smoking has a direct effect on the skin, leaving prominent lines and wrinkles, visible bony contours, gray and atrophied skin, and blotchy discoloration. Smoking causes a narrowing of the blood vessels in the outermost layers of the skin, which results in impaired blood flow to the skin. It also inhibits the production of collagen, thereby weakening the structural support of the epidermis and causing the development of fine lines and wrinkles, and skin that begins to sag years before it should. Even the facial expressions you make while smoking, such as pursing your lips when inhaling, contribute to fine lines and permanent wrinkles over a period of time.

Smoking and sun exposure are synergistic. This means that those individuals who smoke and have years of sun exposure will have worse skin damage than someone who just smokes or just stays out in the sun. As we explain further in this chapter, both smoking and sun exposure are risk factors that you can control — and we recommend addressing both behaviors to slow down premature skin aging.

Smoking Triples the Risk of Skin Cancer

Smoking more than triples your risk of developing squamous cell carcinoma, a serious form of skin cancer. Researchers believe that smoking may damage skin tissue DNA, resulting in errant cell growth.

Facial expressions. Common facial expressions such as frowning, squinting, smiling, and laughing trigger small muscle contractions that, over time, contribute to the development of wrinkles around the eyes and mouth. If you sleep on your stomach or side, you may be increasing the likelihood of permanent creases or wrinkles by the way you rest your face on the pillow. (Sleep on your back to avoid creasing or wrinkling the skin.)

Are You at Risk for Premature Skin Aging?

Risk factors are those lifestyle habits or histories that put you at greater likelihood of a particular condition. For instance, we know that obesity and a sedentary lifestyle increase the risk of diabetes and cardiovascular disease. A diet low in calcium can increase the risk of osteoporosis (thin bones), with subsequent fractures. But there are also specific factors that increase premature skin aging. Some of these may be inherited, such as a family history of premature wrinkling of skin, rosacea (an acne-like condition with rough, reddened skin), or even the predisposition for skin cancer. Other key risk factors include a less than healthy lifestyle, such as a diet devoid of fruits and vegetables, and smoking cigarettes, among others.

No matter what they are, risk factors often do their damage in silence. In other words, even if you don't have any noticeable fine lines,

Environmental Influence on Skin Aging

The environment means anything that is not genetic. Some environmental factors that affect skin aging include:

- Diet
- Air
- Water
- Ultraviolet (UV) radiation
- Health and illness (including stress)

deep wrinkles, or skin damage right now, if you do have any of the risk factors we discuss, it is only a matter of time before you will notice visible signs. The good news is that early recognition of skin-aging risk factors and personal action to change the ones you can control will help revitalize your skin and delay or even reverse the wrinkles and thin, translucent skin associated with premature skin aging.

While it is common for women over forty to have fine lines, wrinkles, and other visible signs of skin aging, the actual process begins much earlier. In fact, the stage is set for skin aging as early as childhood, when the cumulative effect of photodamage begins to take its toll. Consider a newborn's skin and then compare this with that of a preschooler whose face is sprinkled with dark freckles. Babies are not born with splotchy or freckled skin. Freckles are caused by the same process as that which produces sunburn, and people with a predisposition to freckles may be especially susceptible to skin cancer. Exposure to the sun has already begun to damage the quality of the young child's skin. That's why it is so important to know your personal risk factors and prevent early skin damage. You can also protect your children's or grandchildren's skin health by encouraging them to take responsibility for their skin at a time when they can make a difference in preventing photodamage.

No matter what her age, every woman's experience with skin aging is different. Some risk factors are stage-specific, such as pregnancy, which often causes increased hyperpigmentation (melasma).

After pregnancy, the hyperpigmentation may not resolve entirely, leaving the skin spotted and blotchy. As you age, other factors become more prevalent, such as the decline of the hormone estrogen with menopause or the increased risk of precancerous lesions with age and/or sun damage. The good news is that the more risk factors you address and control, the healthier your skin can be.

Earlier in this chapter (page 23), you took a self-assessment to find out your skin age. Now let's take a similar look at four of our clients, their real age and skin age, their personal risk factors for premature skin aging, and their resulting skin conditions. As we move into the Beyond Botox program, you will see how the various steps and specific strategies work to address these risk factors, resulting in sexy, ageless skin.

Client's name: Kim
Real age: 48
Skin age: 54
Risk factors: History of deprivation dieting, cigarette smoking, sun damage
Skin condition: Fine lines, wrinkles, age spots, blotchy complexion

---

Howard met forty-eight-year-old Kim while introducing a new line of B. Kamins, Chemist, cosmeceuticals at a spa in Newport Beach, California. While Howard was demonstrating the topical lotions to spa clientele, this mother of three asked him for help in diminishing the fine lines and wrinkles on her skin. Kim said she had smoked cigarettes since college days and spent most weekends of her life soaking up the California sun while playing tennis or walking the sandy white beaches on the coast. She also had a history of very-low-calorie dieting and was about ten pounds underweight. Kim's skin was extremely thin around her eyes and cheeks, causing it to appear almost transparent. Her neck was tan, and it was clear that the sun had etched deep wrinkles in her skin. Kim said that if she did not wear a heavy foundation, you could see tiny red and blue splotches on her cheeks.

> **Client's name:** Sara
> **Real age:** 53
> **Skin age:** 53
> **Risk factors:** Menopause
> **Skin condition:** Dry skin, loss of subcutaneous fat, fine lines, some wrinkles

Sara went through a natural menopause in her early fifties. In an e-mail to me, she said she had experienced an easy transition without annoying symptoms, but now she was undergoing dramatic skin changes, particularly extremely dry skin that was itchy and blotchy with patches of dark pigmentation. While Sara had taken excellent care of her skin, used sunscreen daily, had a healthy diet, and never smoked cigarettes, she said her skin was now thinner and more transparent, and the tiny laugh lines looked as if "someone had ironed my skin in folds." Topical creams worked temporarily to reduce dryness, but within an hour or two of applying them, Sara said, her skin was dry and flaking again. This made it difficult to wear foundation or powder, as the topical cream changed the color of her makeup, and the powder caked in the creases on her face.

> **Client's name:** Marnie
> **Real age:** 43
> **Skin age:** 49
> **Risk factors:** Rosacea, excessive exercise, low body weight
> **Skin condition:** Redness around nose and cheeks, facial spider veins (telangiectasia)

When traveling to New York City to give a talk on aging skin, I met forty-three-year-old Marnie. This vivacious sales manager said she was having problems managing her rosacea, which had started abruptly in her midthirties. Rosacea, an acneiform disorder that is common in middle-aged and older adults, is characterized by the vascular dilation of the central face (the nose, cheek, eyelids, and forehead) and inflammatory lesions (papules, pustules, cysts, and nodules). An avid exerciser, Marnie said she spent hours each week out of doors, running, hiking, boating, or bike riding. But the combination of sun and wind had irritated her already sensitive and inflamed skin, causing flushing on her cheeks most of the time. Marnie also had tiny red spider veins (telangiectasia) on her cheeks and the sides of her nose.

Client's name: Janis
Real age: 36
Skin age: 46
Risk factors: Vegan diet, sun damage
Skin condition: Acne, pitting, flaking, early wrinkling

Janis, a vegan, had not eaten any animal products for more than fifteen years, since college days. Initially, she e-mailed me to commend me for our company policy on not testing our products on animals. But while Janis was passionate about the animal rights cause, she was less passionate about taking care of herself and getting adequate nourishment.

Janis said that during her late twenties, she got acne for the first time. While acne is prevalent among adolescents, the number of patients over the age of twenty-five with either late-onset or persistent acne is increasing, with acne affecting 8 percent of twenty-five to thirty-four-year-olds and 3 percent of thirty-five to forty-four-year-olds. Janis still had numerous papules and pustules (mainly facial) and mild scarring.

Living on a steady diet of lentils, brown rice, and a few select fruits and vegetables, Janis was also underweight. Her limited diet was missing some key skin nutrients, such as marine omega-3 fatty acids to counter inflammation, essential fatty acids to replenish much-needed oils, and adequate calcium and magnesium to keep her bones and teeth strong.

Janis said she volunteered at an aquarium on weekends and had a lengthy history of sun damage. In fact, she felt that her skin age was at least ten years older than her chronological age.

Taking Control

Perhaps you are surprised to see how specific environmental factors and lifestyle habits influenced skin aging with Kim, Sara, Marnie, and Janis. Don't be! Skin aging is a natural process, but many women simply accept the fine lines and wrinkles that are associated with premature skin aging. And we now realize that skin aging can be greatly accelerated — or delayed — depending on many of the choices we make. For example, women who avoided sun damage over the years tend to look years younger than peers the same age. Likewise, women who avoided cigarette smoke and consistently ate a healthful diet filled with antioxidant-rich fruits and vegetables usually have younger-looking skin than those who have a lengthy history of smoking and a diet filled with processed or junk foods.

Howard recalls meeting twin sisters Mary Anne and Caroline, who approached him after a talk he gave to a women's group in Atlanta, Georgia. The women said they were "fiftyish," but Mary Anne's skin easily looked ten years older than her sister's did. As the women shared with Howard some of their skin-aging risk factors, it became apparent why these women looked so different even though they were the exact same age and had the same genetic heritage.

Here are a few of the risk factors they mentioned:

Mary Anne

1. Smoker (thirty years)
2. Lengthy history of sunbathing
3. Underweight
4. History of very-low-calorie diets
5. Disordered sleep
6. Two basal cell carcinomas removed

Caroline

1. Nonsmoker
2. Rarely went out in the sun
3. Normal weight
4. Pescetarian (vegetarian and some fish)
5. Seven hours of sleep nightly
6. No signs of skin cancer or precancerous lesions

It is quite apparent from these lists why Mary Anne's skin age was ten years older than her twin sister's. Sure, your genes can keep you healthy and looking young up to a point. But there will be a time for most women when environmental factors and lifestyle habits take over, and those are the skin-aging risk factors you can identify right now and start to change.

I believe that all women can take charge of skin-aging risk factors and be the guardians of their own skin. That means making informed decisions regarding early detection, prevention, and treatment of skin conditions to keep it healthy. While treating skin problems is critical, especially in the early stages when treatment works best, there is a compelling case supported by a host of scientific data that the prevention of any skin conditions — including signs of premature aging — should be the primary goal. That said, there is *no mystery* to having sexy, ageless skin. The more risk factors you have, the greater the chance of premature skin aging. However, the sooner you start to control — and change — your risk factors, the more radiant your skin will look as you age. To help you control risk factors, I've given detailed information about these risks and ways to reverse them in our Beyond Botox seven-step program.

How the Beyond Botox Seven-Step Lifestyle Program Can Help

Maybe you've had the same skin care regimen since you were a teenager. Maybe you're seeing the first early signs of aging skin in the mirror every morning. Maybe you're getting distressed that your old products and tricks just don't seem to be working anymore. Maybe you're feeling desperate to know that you're doing something — everything possible! — to keep your skin looking vibrant and healthy.

Having sexy, ageless skin isn't vain. It's important — to your self-esteem, to your relationships, to your career, really to every part of your life, especially in our highly competitive, youth-oriented society. Consciously or unconsciously, we judge each other by our complexion and the way we look. Women today experience loss of self-esteem and even feelings of anxiety and depression when their skin ages prematurely. Aged skin appearance is associated with discrimination in the workplace and even in relationships. That's why I believe it is important to be aware of the emotional side of this issue, so you can take proactive measures to stop premature skin aging before it affects other parts of your life.

Is there an easy answer to the inevitable and relentless intrinsic and extrinsic aging of the skin? Probably not. But there are excellent daily solutions to reverse or slow some of the changes related to both chronological and environmental aging. Over time, these daily strategies will result in healthier, younger-looking skin that makes you feel good about yourself.

In the next chapter, I want to introduce you to the healing effects of specific ingredients you may find in your cosmeceuticals. With a greater understanding of the reparative ingredients in your moisturizer, face wash, night cream, masque, and more, as well as ingredients that might irritate or even damage your skin, I believe that any woman can actively prevent problems that cause her skin to look old before its time.

Chapter 3

What's in Your Medicine Cabinet?

Selecting the Right Products for Your Skin Type

Tired of looking at the visible laugh lines that greet you when you apply your makeup each day, you decide to check out the latest cosmeceuticals at a nearby body boutique. As you peruse the various anti-aging therapies, you notice that the promises are similar: erasing fine lines and wrinkles, boosting collagen in the skin, and restoring a youthful glow. But which products are most effective and safe? Do you choose organic or natural, a cream or a lotion? How concentrated should the ingredients be? Most important, is there any science that substantiates the advertising claims?

Finally, after listening to a persuasive salesclerk tell of customers who look "decades younger" after using her company's products, you select a moisturizer and toner and feel okay about your purchase . . . until you get home and read the package insert and find that both products are heavily fragranced with flower essence — and you are highly allergic to pollen and fragrance. What's a woman to do when it comes to finding trusted products and effective ingredients for healthy, ageless skin?

*　　*　　*

As a pharmaceutical chemist, I am often dismayed at the unrealistic promises made by cosmetics companies. Why, I wonder, would they select ingredients that are known to be ineffective, or fragranced ingredients that trigger allergies in some women, and put them into popular skin care products? I believe that women should understand the content of their moisturizer, scrub, eye cream, or anti-aging therapy and know whether the ingredients work to rejuvenate the skin or do more harm than good by causing rough, splotchy complexions. I believe that with a better understanding of the ingredients in skin care products, combined with the implementation of the practical lifestyle strategies discussed in our Beyond Botox seven-step program, any woman, *no matter what her age,* can enjoy sexy, ageless skin for years to come.

In the early 1990s, I asked my scientific staff to begin investigating the symptoms of hormone-deprived skin in both perimenopausal (the two to eight years preceding menopause) and menopausal women. Several of my staff members groaned. Perhaps this request seemed somewhat frivolous to them, but it was not to me. For months, I'd been spending my days (and many nights) in the lab, researching and developing products that were helping others' skin to look beautiful. But back at home, my wife, Mildred, also had an urgent need — a better treatment for her aging skin.

Healthy Skin on the Home Front

I am blessed to have been married to the same woman for more than forty years. When I first met Mildred, she enjoyed sunbathing and spent hours outdoors perfecting her summer tan. Like many women in the 1960s and 1970s, she used a "tan booster" — an aluminum tanning reflector that angled the sun's rays directly onto her skin. Of course, hindsight tells us that this was just about the worst thing a young person could do to her skin. Although Mildred's summer tans faded as fall approached, the sun damage from those early years stayed with her.

When she was in her thirties and forties, Mildred repeatedly told me that her skin and hair care products did not work effectively. She often asked, "Ben, can't you make me moisturizers for my dry skin that won't make me break out?" Or, "Won't you make me a rich conditioner that gives my hair more bounce and luster but does not make it oily?" By the early 1990s, Mildred began to notice new and different skin changes that coincided with the onset of menopause and the rapid decline of the hormone estrogen. These changes included thinner and much drier skin, increased bruising, and uneven pigmentation. As we've already learned, these symptoms are extremely common effects of menopause, but it was still tough for Mildred to accept the skin changes she saw in the mirror each day.

At the time, there was little interest among other scientists or cosmetics companies in developing creams specifically for women at menopause. The terms *menopause* and *hormone replacement therapy* were often whispered among women but never spoken in public — much less in a laboratory. I started reading everything I could find on the topic . . . which wasn't much. I found a marked scarcity of scientific studies involving menopausal skin — in fact, as was the case with most health studies at the time, the main dermatological research was done on men, not women. It became clear to me, however, that women had unique needs and symptoms when it comes to the life cycle changes in their skin. Something had to be done, and I was on a mission.

Isolating the Healing Ingredients

Although perplexed as to how to assist my wife in resolving her new skin concerns, I was committed to discovering some way to alleviate her symptoms. During that time, I accompanied some friends on a winter ice-fishing trip in northern Canada. While there, I noticed that the hardy maple trees (*Acer saccharum*) surrounding the icy lakes survived and even thrived in Canada's cold, unforgiving climate. I was greatly puzzled and impressed by the resiliency of the maple trees, and when I returned to my lab, I acquired a small quantity of raw maple sap for analysis.

As the specific compounds from the maple extract were analyzed, I again pored over the medical literature, this time searching for scientific evidence on the benefits of maple extract in topical applications. I also had lengthy discussions with my professional colleagues and some of the finest researchers in North America. Finally, I concluded that the maple isolate was a material that just might be able to help treat the very complex changes that occur when skin ages. Maple isolate was well-suited for use in a topical preparation, which I was convinced could address the short- and long-term needs associated with my wife's dramatic skin changes at menopause.

Once I purified the maple isolate into an all-natural, nontoxic, skin-penetrating additive, I realized that I had a very useful ingredient that could meet the specialized skin care needs of women of all ages. The maple isolate was filled with pure antioxidants that had anti-wrinkling action and that would infuse the outer layer of the epidermis to help fight free radicals, the highly reactive and unstable molecules that are thought to damage cellular DNA and are linked to diseases and the aging process. It also contained anti-wrinkle amino-peptides and AHA malic acid. The total effect of the preparation was nontoxic, anti-aging, and even moisturizing by attracting water molecules from the environment. This was a perfect physiological humectant, which I'm proud to say was researched and developed in our labs.

Recognizing that there are multiple skin changes during menopause, I created a unique topical cream for my wife using this maple isolate, as well as other appropriate ingredients to treat the multiple skin changes directly related to hormone deprivation. When I finally brought the lab sample home, Mildred told me how cool and refreshing it felt on her warm face — calming the redness, itching, and irritation caused by hot flashes. A few weeks later, her friends were commenting that her skin looked firmer and younger, and that the tiny lines and wrinkles on her face were greatly diminished. Mildred was thrilled with the compound and the adulation from her peers — and that made me feel good too.

What This Means for Your Skin

Today I smile when I think of the story of how my discovery virtually "saved my marriage." But in addition to making my home life a whole lot smoother, this work marked the beginning of a passionate project, redirecting my work and inspiring my life's mission — to better understand the physiological, biochemical, and architectural skin changes that occur as women age. Since that time, I have continued to create hundreds of innovative healing formulas to treat myriad skin problems for men, women, and children.

But what I *don't* want is for this book to be an advertisement for my products — or for any particular product. A significant part of our Beyond Botox seven-step program involves the various lifestyle changes that will make a dramatic difference in your skin's appearance. But the right cosmeceutical ingredients, applied correctly and in conjunction with other lifestyle choices, *can* make a significant difference in your skin's appearance. What this chapter is meant to do is give you a better understanding of the most effective ingredients used in cosmeceuticals so you can make a personal plan to develop beautiful, ageless skin for yourself — by reading the labels and making smart choices about what the right ingredients can do for your skin.

What Are Cosmeceuticals?

In even the recent past, women had to resort to homespun techniques like oleomargarine, honey, and lemon juice to keep their skin looking young and supple as they aged. Luckily, today a dizzying array of drugs, cosmetics, and cosmeceuticals exists to help. A product is classified as a drug if it is used to prevent or treat a disease and a cosmetic if it is used for enhancement and beautification of appearance. A cosmeceutical is a hybrid of these two — it's a cosmetic product that has druglike benefits. Interestingly, there are few sharp dividing lines between drugs and cosmetics, and many preparations are classified as cosmeceutical hybrids.

In my laboratories, I formulate cosmeceuticals that treat multiple skin problems, using ingredients that have numerous reparative and anti-aging properties. Every year, chemists like myself are learning more about biotechnology and gaining a better understanding of the physiology and structure of the skin, and as a result we are able to produce unique skin care preparations that for the first time address and slow many skin-aging symptoms.

The key is to match specific cosmeceuticals to each specific type of skin. As my wife (and many of my clients) have found, if you don't match your skin with the right product, the results can be disappointing, even dire. Over the past decade, Howard and I have talked with literally hundreds of women just like you who were desperately seeking anti-aging solutions but who were clueless about various products' ingredients and effectiveness when applied to their skin.

One of these women was Candace, who was in her early forties. Candace said that in preparation for her niece's wedding, she had started a "get back in shape" regimen. Not only had she lost twelve pounds by watching her diet and exercising daily, but her blood pressure was lower and she was learning to take time for herself each day to relax and enjoy life's journey.

Wanting her skin to look as good as she felt, Candace had asked her primary care physician for Renova, a prescription formulation similar to Retin-A. She said that her best friend had used Renova for more than a year and the difference in the skin appearance was quite noticeable. These creams slough off the skin's dead surface cells, thicken the healthy cells, and increase the production of collagen. All of these actions result in the skin appearing suppler and less wrinkled.

Unfortunately, after using Renova for less than two weeks, Candace (like many women I have seen) had dramatic negative side effects, including dryness, inflammation, redness, and peeling. She complained that her physician had not warned her that the side effects could be so debilitating, and she was forced to cancel her wedding trip because of the extreme irritation, redness, and peeling.

Jennifer is another example of a woman who was desperate for younger-looking skin but simply did not know which ingredients to use, especially during menopause. This fifty-one-year-old mother of two teenagers worked as a part-time legal assistant in Scottsdale, Arizona, where the average high temperature in July is 104 degrees (F) with relatively low humidity. She said that for most of her adult life, her skin had been quite normal, even in Arizona's hot, dry climate, so she had really never thought about what topical skin care products to use.

As if overnight, Jennifer said, her skin became ultradry and scaly, with small crusty patches on her cheeks and arms, and nothing seemed to help resolve it. Upon questioning, I learned that Jennifer had been using a light-textured daytime moisturizer that she "borrowed" from her teenage daughter. Because of Arizona's climate combined with her own dramatic decline in hormones, I felt that Jennifer needed to be much more aggressive in caring for her skin to combat its new ultradry state.

I suggested that Jennifer change her skin care regimen to include a heavy-duty moisturizer that contained ingredients such as petrolatum, urea, sodium lactate, and squalane, along with a sunblock. I also suggested that she change her skin cleanser, which she also "borrowed" from her teenager, as it was overly efficient in removing natural skin oils, resulting in an even drier complexion. At nighttime, I recommended that Jennifer use a concentrated, multipurpose, antioxidant barrier-repair cream that contained petrolatum, ceramides, and sodium hyaluronate.

Three weeks later, Jennifer phoned to say that she now saw a definite improvement in her skin texture and realized that her life-long skin care products were simply inadequate for her menopausal dry skin.

Hope or Hype?

Under the 1938 Federal Food, Drug, and Cosmetic Act, cosmetics are defined as "articles intended to be rubbed, poured, sprinkled, or sprayed on, introduced into, or otherwise applied to the human body or any part thereof for cleansing, beautifying, promoting attractiveness, or altering the appearance." Drugs are defined as products intended for treating or preventing disease and affecting the structure or any function of the body.

All drugs must undergo a premarket review and approval by the FDA, but cosmetics do not have this requirement. Though the FDA considers cosmeceuticals to be cosmetics, many of these products have actions similar to those of drugs, as they effectively prevent skin changes and some skin diseases with their active ingredients.

How Will Cosmeceuticals Help My Skin?

Unlike the skin lotions of years past that simply smelled like roses, left the skin feeling soft, and accomplished very little, today's cosmeceuticals have numerous additional benefits including anti-wrinkle, anti-aging, and wound-healing. There are no magic ingredients that can virtually turn back the clock, but understanding the function of the most effective ingredients and how they work on the skin allows you to select specific cosmeceuticals that best meet your skin's needs — and toss those products that are ineffective or even irritating. Let's look at some of the "behind the scenes" action of these ingredients and how they function at a cellular level to give healing benefits to the skin.

Activate Cellular Repair

Some ingredients used in cosmeceuticals are biologically active, which means they function at the level of the cell. These ingredients play a role in regulating skin cell communication by giving instructions as to how the various bodily structures are supposed to function. This cellular communication is part of all repair processes leading to natural healing and involves diverse biological factors that activate cell repair mechanisms. This happens when specific molecules bind to their appropriate receptors in the manner of a puzzle, where only the right piece can fit into a certain spot.

Cell receptors are specialized sites on the cell membrane. The retinoids (page 47), which are derivatives of vitamin A, are good examples of cell receptor activators, meaning they are able to bind or connect to a specific site on the cell membrane and communicate with the cell. The retinoid receptors play a role in skin cell differentiation, organization, and pigmentation.

Restore Hydration

One of the primary roles of the skin is to act as a barrier to protect muscles, tendons, and internal organs and structures from environmental damage and infection. For the skin to maintain an optimal barrier function, its hydration level is very important. A primary function of effective cosmeceutical ingredients is to maintain or restore the skin's optimal hydration level. Moisturizers based on petrolatum, glycerin, urea, sodium PCA, or the B. Kamins Bio-Maple or similar compounds provide the skin with immediate hydration, which is crucial, especially for dry and sensitive skin types and aging skin.

Promote Exfoliation

Cosmeceutical products often contain a low concentration of skin-exfoliating agents, such as glycolic acid, lactic acid (alpha hydroxy acid [AHA]), and/or salicylic acid (beta hydroxy acid [BHA]), which promote the shedding of dead skin cells to maintain the skin's youthful and smooth complexion. Skin-exfoliating agents work very effectively in the loosening of the dead cells of the stratum corneum and on acne-prone skin with plugged pores and dry, flaky skin.

Fight Oxidation

Antioxidants are among the natural defense mechanisms that protect skin against additional oxidative (aging) processes. Antioxidant creams help to combat potentially harmful wrinkle-causing free radicals, which are often generated after sun exposure. Free radicals trigger an inflammatory response that many believe leads to skin aging. The use of topical antioxidants that minimize the action of free radical scavengers can slow down skin aging.

Topical antioxidant ingredients include vitamin E, vitamin A, vitamin C, green tea, and hundreds of other compounds that contain polyphenols or related ingredients. The duration of the antioxidant action on the skin is relatively short, and repeat applications of antioxidant preparations are necessary.

Decrease Inflammation

Inflammation is a reaction of the body to injury or to an infectious, allergic, or chemical irritation. The symptoms of skin inflammation include redness, swelling, heat, and pain resulting from dilation of the blood vessels in the affected part. Many topical cosmeceuticals contain therapeutically active ingredients that can cause inflammatory reactions such as tingling or tightening and/or visual signs such as redness or rash. Anti-inflammatory ingredients are thus incorporated into these preparations to counteract the unwanted reactions and to allow the chemist to use more therapeutically active ingredients with fewer incidences of side effects.

I usually add niacinamide or a botanical extract such as bisabolol (from chamomile) to decrease skin inflammation and protect the cells from oxidation. I also add vitamins like tocopherol acetate or ascorbic acid phosphate, both of which have antioxidative properties. Sometimes I add synthetic biologically active peptides such as acetyl-hexapeptide-3 (Argireline) that mimic natural molecules and have therapeutic properties.

Commonly Used Anti-Inflammatory Ingredients

1. Alpha lipoic acid
2. Beta-glucan (polysaccharide derived from yeast)
3. Bisabolol (chamomile extract)
4. Canola oil *(Brassica napus)*
5. Green tea extract *(Camellia sinensis)*
6. Licorice extract (glycyrrhetic acid)
7. Oat extract *(Avena sativa)*
8. Soy extract *(Glycine soja)*
9. Vitamin E (tocopheral)
10. Vitamin C (L-ascorbic acid)

Increase Photoprotection

Photoprotection is a fancy way of saying sunscreen. It is imperative for anti-aging cosmeceutical treatments to include sunscreens. Photoprotection is dependent on the pigmentation level of the skin, which is regulated through UVA-induced melanin production. It is vital to protect the skin from sun rays when spending time outside, since UVA sun rays also cause irreversible collagen and elastin degradation, leading to premature skin aging.

What Cosmeceuticals Should I Use?

By understanding your skin aging risks, discussed in chapter 2, and specific skin problems, you can find the most helpful healing ingredients for your skin. With greater knowledge of how each ingredient works, you can read the labels on your skin care products and identify those ingredients that may work well, may not work at all, or may even cause irritation or damage your skin.

In the seven-step program (chapters 4 through 10), I discuss in depth the various skin types and specific skin problems, including the causes, signs and symptoms, and ingredients to use for prevention and treatment of these problems. For now, I want to help you to understand which ingredients I use in cosmeceuticals to help resolve different skin problems.

Review the following common skin problems and checkmark those that are most troublesome to you. Then read the list of ingredients that I add to formulations in my laboratory to combat each of these problems. You'll find more information on the specific function of each ingredient in the sidebar on page 50.

1. Itchy skin

Beyond Botox recommendations: Petrolatum, menthyl lactate, bisabolol, allantoin, and/or zinc oxide

2. Dry skin

Beyond Botox recommendations: Petrolatum, squalane, urea, oleic acid, lecithin, Bio-Maple, ceramides, hyaluronic acid, cholesterol, and/or sodium lactate

3. Normal skin

Beyond Botox recommendations: Petrolatum, glycerin, hyaluronic acid, phospholipids, and/or squalane

4. Flaky skin

Beyond Botox recommendations: Petrolatum, salicylic acid, mineral oil, squalane, and/or safflower oil

5. Oily skin

Beyond Botox recommendations: Salicylic acid, glycolic acid, lactic acid, and/or witch hazel

6. Adult acne

Beyond Botox recommendations: Benzoyl peroxide, salicylic acid, resorcinol, azelaic acid, and/or retinoids (Rx)

7. Allergic skin

Beyond Botox recommendations: Petrolatum, glycerin, sodium PCA, sodium hyaluronate, and/or urea

8. Wrinkles around the eye area

Beyond Botox recommendations: Hyaluronic acid, petrolatum, squalane, soya proteins, amino oligoelements, and/or ceramides

9. Dark circles under the eyes

Beyond Botox recommendations: Vitamin K, silica, hesperetin, and/or zinc oligopeptide

10. Laugh lines

Beyond Botox recommendations: Ceramides, petrolatum, phospholipids, soya sterols, and/or cholesterol

11. Lip lines (vertical)

Beyond Botox recommendations: Petrolatum, paraffin, squalane, and/or carnauba wax

12. Sagging, loose skin

Beyond Botox recommendations: Soya protein, soya sterols, mulberry extract, phospholipids, and/or ceramides

13. Reddened rosacea-type skin

Beyond Botox recommendations: Bisabolol, squalane, Bio-Maple, glycerin, niaciamide, and/or micronized zinc oxide

14. Sun spots or age spots

Beyond Botox recommendations: Hydroquinone, kojic acid, salicylic acid, and/or vitamin C ester

15. Sun-damaged skin

Beyond Botox recommendations: AHAs, salicylic acid, ceramides, Bio-Maple, phytosterols, sodium PCA, and/or mucopolysaccharides

What Are the Retinoids?

The retinoids (retinoic acid and tretinoin), also antioxidants, are a family of fat-soluble compounds that play an important role in cell division, eyesight, reproduction, and bone growth. Topically, retinol is one of the most active forms of vitamin A and is found in whole milk and fortified foods. It can be converted to retinoic acid and other forms of vitamin A. Vitamin A acid (tretinoin) is a prescription medication in cream or gel form that is used to help improve sun-damaged skin, reduce coarse and fine wrinkles, and normalize areas of skin discoloration.

What Are Alpha Hydroxy Acids?

Alpha hydroxy acids (AHAs) are a commonly used ingredient in skin care products. AHAs work by promoting exfoliation in the outer layer of skin, resulting in a healthier-looking, clearer complexion. Products containing AHAs became wildly popular in the 1990s — not only were the AHAs moisturizing and exfoliating, but they were naturally derived from citrus fruit, apples, pears, and milk. Because the ingredients were natural, people felt good about putting AHAs on their face.

AHAs are one of the safest methods of skin renewal. Still, their effectiveness depends on the type and concentration of the AHA, the pH (acidity), and other ingredients in the topical product. The AHAs used most often in cosmetics include glycolic acid and lactic acid, although there are many others (see list below), and many AHAs are used in combination.

If your product contains one of the following ingredients, it contains alpha hydroxy acids (AHA):

- glycolic acid
- lactic acid
- citric acid
- malic acid
- tartaric acid
- glycolic acid + ammonium glycolate
- alpha hydroxyethanoic acid + ammonium alpha hydroxy-ethanoate
- alpha hydroxyoctanoic acid
- alpha hydroxycaprylic acid
- hydroxycaprylic acid
- mixed fruit acid
- triple fruit acid
- tri-alpha hydroxy fruit acids
- sugar cane extract
- alpha hydroxy and botanical complex
- L-alpha hydroxy acid
- glycomer in cross-linked fatty acids alpha nutrium

Natural or Synthetic?

Whenever I give talks to groups about a chemist's perspective on cosmeceuticals and skin aging, invariably I am asked whether a product is "natural." I acknowledge that natural ingredients are assumed to be safer and healthier for both humans and the environment; I also know that there is no one definition of a natural product. As a chemist, I have a healthy respect — and disrespect — for natural ingredients.

Some natural materials have been around for thousands of years, and there is a perception that these are safer than man-made ingredients. Even so, natural materials need to be closely scrutinized to prevent unwanted effects before incorporating them into topical preparations for the skin.

Coming from the pharmaceutical world, I also recognize that the vast majority of therapeutic agents that save lives are synthesized in scientific laboratories and come from the first ninety-two elements of the periodic table. In reality, very few of these agents are derived from "natural sources."

Knowledge Is Key to Reversing Skin Aging

As you've no doubt already experienced, choosing the best skin care products (though important) can only take you so far. Healthy, youthful skin requires a healthy, youthful lifestyle. That said, I believe that every woman — no matter what her age — should rethink her approach to skin care, especially as modern lifestyle habits such as deprivation dieting, cigarette smoking, and tanning trigger a heightened vulnerability to premature aging of the skin.

I urge you after reading this chapter to gather your various cosmeceuticals and read the product labels just as you do the labels on prepackaged foods. Carefully compare the ingredients listed on the labels to the ingredients explained in this chapter to see if you are using the most effective healing products for your skin problems.

The steps you take starting right now to reverse aging skin need not be radical, time consuming, or expensive. Instead, armed with the latest scientific studies and a chemist's expert advice, you can make informed choices tailored to meet your specific skin care needs and enjoy sexy, ageless skin for years to come. Part II of this book, the Beyond Botox seven-step program, will show you how.

Understanding Ingredients

Now that you have an idea of the exact ingredients I use in formulating cosmeceuticals, I want to explain what these effective ingredients *do* when applied to the skin. I believe that it is important to give you an honest appraisal of these ingredients, as they are so commonly used in lotions, creams, and ointments.

Allantonin is extracted from plants or obtained as a by-product of uric acid. It is used in cosmetic preparations as an anti-irritant ingredient to soothe and reduce inflammation.

Amino oligoelements, a class of compounds that includes minerals such as zinc or copper linked to amino acid peptides, are used as healing, anti-aging ingredients in cosmeceuticals.

Azelaic acid, a component of grains such as wheat, rye, and barley, is used as a treatment for acne and in some anti-aging skin preparations.

Benzoyl peroxide, an antibacterial agent with a drying effect on skin, is most effective for inflammatory acne consisting of pustules (sores), papules (bumps), and comedons (whiteheads). When using this ingredient, always wear an oil-free sunscreen to protect your skin.

Bio-Maple is a natural physiological humectant/moisturizer that includes mono- and polysaccharides, amino acids, polyphenols, malic acid, isoflavones, and minerals (calcium, potassium, and phosphorous), among other plant growth substances. Bio-Maple is nontoxic and contains a mixture of water-attracting molecules, nutrients, naturally occurring AHA, anti-wrinkle antioxidants, and moisturizing anti-aging amino acid peptides.

Carnauba wax is a natural wax obtained from the leaves of palm trees, used primarily as a thickening and film-forming agent in cosmetic preparations.

Ceramides (sphingolipids and phospholipids), naturally occurring skin lipids that are part of the skin's outer structure, are important for the skin's water-retention capacity.

Cholesterol, a lipid naturally found in human skin oil, has a water-binding capacity and is very important in repairing normal skin barrier function.

Glycerin (glycerol) is a moisturizing ingredient that works best in a humid environment.

(continued)

Glycolic acid, an alpha hydroxy acid (AHA), is used in milder strengths in over-the-counter exfoliants and moisturizers, at 20 percent or 30 percent at spas for a more intense peeling effect, and at 70 percent solution for physicians who do skin peeling.

Hydroquinone, commonly used as a skin-lightening agent, is applied topically in the treatment of melasma (chloasma, or mask of pregnancy), freckles, and senile lentigines (brown spots, liver spots). It is important to wear a sunscreen when using hydroquinone.

Kojic acid, a by-product from the fermentation of rice, is used in skin-lightening formulations for inhibiting melanin production.

Lecithin, a phospholipid found in the membranes of plant and animal cells, is used as an emollient and water-binding agent in cosmetic preparations.

Menthyl lactate, a derivative of menthol, is used as a cooling agent in topical creams and lotions.

Mineral oil, also called liquid paraffin, liquid petrolatum, white mineral oil, and white paraffin oil, is used to prevent skin drying and irritation.

Mucopolysaccharides, a large class of ingredients known as glycosaminoglycans, are excellent moisturizing ingredients because of their water-binding capacity. Mucopolysaccharides include hyaluronic acid, naturally found in skin tissue.

Mulberry extract is a botanical with both astringent (skin-tightening) and antibacterial properties.

Oleic acid, an essential fatty acid found in animal and vegetable oils, is used in skin creams to help restore normal skin barrier function.

Peptides have anti-inflammatory properties and are used in the treatment of skin wounds and as skin-firming and wrinkle-reducing agents in cosmeceutical preparations.

Petrolatum is a moisturizing agent that serves as a base for other ingredients in cosmeceutical products and helps prevent transepidermal water loss (TEWL) due to its occlusive (film-forming) properties.

Phytosterols are cholesterol-like molecules found in plants such as soy and wheat, and are used as emollients in topical creams and lotions.

Salicylic acid is used in topical acne preparations and treatments for psoriasis, dandruff, viral warts, and corns and calluses. Used topically, salicylic acid encourages the removal of dead skin cells.

(continued)

Sodium hyaluronate helps to retain the natural moisture content of the skin better than most ingredients and is extremely safe and nonirritating.

Sodium lactate (from lactic acid) is an excellent moisturizer because of its hygroscopic (water-attracting) humectant properties and also helps to exfoliate dead skin cells.

Sodium pyrrolidone carboxylate (sodium PCA) is a natural moisturizer present in all living cells, but its production decreases with age.

Soya proteins have a tightening effect on the skin and form a very fine moisturizing "film" on the epidermis to help protect skin and minimize the development of wrinkles and surface roughness.

Squalane is a naturally occurring oil found in human skin. This fine emollient does a superb job of keeping skin protected and moisturized.

Urea, a moisturizing ingredient, is commonly used to treat rough, dry skin. Urea has anti-itch actions and, at higher concentrations (10 to 25 percent), acts as a keratolytic (softening and peeling) skin agent.

Vitamin C (ascorbic acid), a water-soluble antioxidant found in fruits and vegetables, is used in its "ester" form as an antioxidant, a skin lightener, and an exfoliant. Because its benefits in topical preparations are somewhat controversial, I usually combine vitamin C with other ingredients when using it in topical preparations.

Vitamin E, a fat-soluble antioxidant found in vegetable oils, nuts, whole grains, and leafy vegetables, is used in creams and lotions as an antioxidant to help protect skin cells against the harmful effects of free radicals and with other emollient materials to treat dry skin and scar tissue.

Witch hazel is a natural extract from the *Hamamelis* plant that is used in cosmetics as an antioxidant, astringent, and tonic due to its tannin content.

PART II:

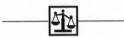

The Beyond Botox 7-Step Program

Now that you know how your skin works, it's time to learn how to start caring for it properly. In the rest of this book, you'll learn the seven most important things you can do to keep your skin sexy and ageless . . . and that it's even possible to turn back the clock and revitalize tired skin. Keep reading to find out how.

Chapter 4

Step #1: Nourish

Feed Your Skin from the Inside Out

Perhaps Zsa Zsa Gabor said it best: "After forty, you have to choose between your fanny and your face."

I'd like to believe that's not the case. But it does speak to one of the most important things I tell people — especially women — who come to me on the quest for younger, sexier skin: although it is vital to be fit and trim to stay healthy and prevent chronic illness, depriving the body of healing nutrients in the quest to be too thin can make one look old, tired, and definitely not sexy.

Through the years in the cosmeceutical industry, I have seen repeatedly that when women starve themselves to be too thin, it ultimately shows on the face. The long-term result will be ultradry skin, sunken eyes and cheeks, fine lines and deep wrinkles, and an overall older-looking appearance. Take our client Nancy, for example, who contacted us for help in "age-proofing" her skin.

This trim, vivacious fifty-one-year-old boutique owner from New Jersey took pride in wearing the same size she had worn in college, some three decades ago. But, though a size two was flattering at age twenty, the years of deprivation dieting it took to stay a size two had taken a toll on Nancy's skin. The skin on her face was almost transparent and extremely wrinkled, with little subcutaneous fat to support it.

Not only did Nancy diet excessively, she'd also smoked cigarettes most of her adult life so she would not snack and could stay thin and energetic. An avid skier, Nancy had ignored applying sunscreen during her frequent trips to the Vermont and Colorado slopes, thinking it was not necessary, as she rarely got sunburned. Recently, a dermatologist removed two precancerous skin lesions from her ear and forehead, and warned her about the extensive sun damage on her face, neck, and arms. Nancy also had fractured her ankle twice over the past year. She said her rheumatologist had diagnosed her with early bone loss, or osteopenia, and said she was at greater risk of more fractures if she did not change her diet.

We talked at length about risk factors for premature skin aging in chapter 2. Let's review Nancy's risk factors for premature skin aging:

- Her age: 51 (menopausal)
- Underweight
- Deprivation dieting
- Cigarette smoking
- Exposure to the sun's ultraviolet radiation

When you add up the risk factors, you have a powerful combination that has resulted in Nancy looking at least ten years older than her biological age. Nancy took our Skin Age Quiz (page 23) and scored 23 out of 30, indicating that the real age of her skin was sixty-one, not fifty-one.

I convinced Nancy that some dietary changes would benefit her skin and help to combat the premature aging caused by the sun, cigarettes, and other risk factors. We also encouraged her to talk to her doctor about the best weight for her height and age. Lauren vowed to start working with a therapy group in New York City for support in stopping cigarettes. I also instructed her in selecting skin care preparations that had healing ingredients such as hyaluronic acid, urea, sodium lactate, squalane, glycerin, petrolatum, sodium PCA, and Bio-Maple compound.

Today, Nancy is at a normal weight for her height and age. She has not smoked in eighteen months and is thrilled that the tiny lines and wrinkles are greatly diminished. Nancy feels younger, sexier, and more alive than she has in years — and friends and colleagues are amazed at her "new" beautiful skin.

*   *   *

For years, experts have recommended special diets to maintain a healthy body — you don't blink an eye when your doctor tells you to cut out butter or red meat to lower your cholesterol. Yet science has been less proactive in identifying the exact foods that are necessary to keep your skin looking healthy and ageless. Many women take the condition of their skin for granted, but I believe you must feed the skin from the inside in order for it to radiate ageless sex appeal on the outside.

Several recent medical studies have revealed a strong connection between certain diets, immune function, and the skin. In fact, researchers are finding that deficiencies of single nutrients can result in increased inflammation, altered immune response, and cell destruction. Scientific findings also indicate that a number of chronic and damaging skin problems such as acne and rosacea are linked to diet either directly or indirectly. These findings have been observed outwardly on the skin — even when the nutritional deficiency is mild.

The good news is this: even moderate changes in your diet can yield significant results in the appearance of your skin. That's why I tell clients that changing their diet is the easiest (and most effective) thing they can do to have an immediate impact on the way their skin looks. As I've said before, I believe that every woman has the potential to look and feel her very best, no matter what her age. The most effective way to enjoy sexy, ageless skin your entire life is to feed your body from the inside out and keep your immune system strong so you stay well.

The Risks of Deprivation Dieting

Most women admit to "deprivation dieting" — defined as consuming fewer than 1,000 to 1,100 calories daily — at some point in their lifetime. But the long-term consequences of this can be severe. Restricting your caloric intake for the long term often results in your body not getting enough dietary protein, and this leads to a breakdown in the healthy function of the immune system.

Deprivation Dieting Can Lead to Chronic Illness

The immune system is your body's healing system and also your natural defense against infection and disease, including cancer. Its main function is to distinguish itself (your bodily system) from nonself (a host of invading germs) through a complex network of antibodies, proteins, and specialized cells. All of these cells have a task, which is to keep you healthy at all costs by attacking and demolishing foreign materials. If some part of this process fails, the immune system itself fails to function as it should, and you get sick — or you suffer with the resulting sallow or dry skin, fine lines and wrinkles, and chronic skin conditions, even skin cancer.

Changes in levels of hormones produced by daily stress can also negatively affect immune function, particularly the nerve cells connecting the brain to other vital organs. The nerve cells are directly involved in making immune system cells, and when stress levels increase, it results in an overproduction of stress hormones that tear down or weaken our immune system . . . and thereby trigger skin aging.

Nancy said that she rarely ate protein and existed on large salads and some bread. But protein is necessary to build and repair body tissue and to fight infection. Too little protein in the diet can lead to symptoms of fatigue, weakness, and poor immunity. The average adult needs forty-five to fifty-five grams of protein a day — even more if you're sick or fighting off a fever or infection. That's the equivalent of five to six ounces of lean meat (say, a typical chicken breast) and two cups of low-fat milk or soy milk per day. Vegetable proteins (legumes, beans, and tofu) are excellent substitutes for animal protein as part of a properly balanced diet.

Deprivation Dieting Can Lead to Acne

Another unpleasant side effect of a low-protein diet — acne. Some recent findings indicate that a highly processed diet that is low in protein may contribute to skin conditions such as acne. Adult acne affects millions of women in their twenties, thirties, and forties, and it's on the rise. Because acne is so common in western nations, yet extremely rare in nonwesternized societies, scientists at the School of Applied Sciences at RMIT University in Melbourne, Australia, questioned whether the acne trigger might be the typical western diet, which includes foods high on the glycemic index such as potatoes, white bread, and pastries. Foods low on the glycemic index (meat, chicken, fish, soy products, and some vegetables) cause a small rise in blood sugar; foods high on the glycemic index (baked potato, starchy foods, desserts) trigger a more dramatic rise, which can influence glucose and endocrine function. After rigorous testing, the team of scientists concluded that eating a diet low on the glycemic index (i.e., higher in protein) can reduce the hormonal fluctuations that cause acne in teenagers and adults.

Deprivation Dieting Can Lead to Weak Bones

Nancy's history of dieting, along with cigarette smoking and being underweight, resulted in early bone loss (osteopenia), with two painful ankle fractures. You may be surprised to hear that someone Nancy's age had early bone loss with fractures, but don't be. Osteopenia is linked to such lifestyle habits as social drinking, lack of calcium in the diet, cigarette smoking, and even drinking excessive amounts of coffee and diet cola. Women who are underweight as a result of deprivation dieting or exercise obsession often experience amenorrhea (absent menstrual periods), even in their twenties or thirties. Because of the important role estrogen plays in keeping bones strong, amenorrhea can lead to early bone loss and even to early menopause, complete with the final cessation of menstrual periods.

Deprivation Dieting Can Lead to Sagging Skin

A history of yo-yo dieting (gaining and losing weight repeatedly) often results in sagging or drooping skin. You might notice this in the folds of skin on your neck after losing weight. Repeatedly gaining and losing weight puts added stress on the skin's elasticity, and your skin won't spring back into its former shape as quickly.

So What *Should* I Eat for Beautiful Skin?

Okay, so I've made my case. Too much dieting and too little protein are bad for your skin. This isn't going to be a book about what you can't do — it's about what you *can* do to promote healthier, younger-looking skin. And I'm here to tell you that eating the right nutrients can make a huge difference in your skin's appearance.

Over the past few years, there has been mounting proof that highly specific nutrients are crucial for slowing down the skin changes associated with aging, and the right nutrients may even

Get Sexy, Ageless Eyes

An eight-year study published in the December 28, 2005, issue of the *Journal of the American Medical Association* confirmed that beta-carotene, vitamins C and E, and zinc appear to lower the risk of macular degeneration, the leading cause of blindness among the elderly in developed countries. In macular degeneration, abnormal blood cells grow in the eye and leak blood and fluid that damage the center of the retina and blur central vision. Sufferers are often unable to read, recognize faces, or drive, and the condition worsens with age.

reverse skin damage. I'll talk about the nutrients you need to add to your diet (I call them skin savers) and discuss what role each can play in protecting your skin from the ravages of time. For example, vitamin C is essential for building collagen in the skin. And selenium-rich foods such as Brazil nuts, tuna, and turkey play a potential role in cancer prevention. These selenium skin savers may also help reduce inflammation associated with acne and rosacea.

But one of the myths we'll be debunking is the idea that eating large amounts of fish — such as the much-touted salmon-heavy diets of other skin care gurus — is good for your skin. As we'll show, though omega-3 fatty acids (such as those found in salmon) are an important part of a healthy diet, eating too much salmon, tuna, and other fish puts you at risk for buildup of injurious toxins, such as mercury, dioxins, and PCB, in the body. We'll offer some smarter, safer ways to get those omega-3 fatty acids into your diet.

Although the individual properties and functions of each nutrient are important, it's the sum of their effectiveness that actually strengthens the immune system, helping to prevent photoaging and promote healthy skin. So at the end of the chapter, we'll give you an eating plan to put all this information together and figure out how to incorporate each of these skin savers into your diet. But first, let's talk about a few of the important vitamins and minerals you should know about as you look at food labels and start to put together your next shopping list.

Boost Your Antioxidants to Combat UV Damage

Skin naturally uses the antioxidants found in fruits, vegetables, and a few other food types to defend itself from damage by UV-induced oxidation. Over time, repeated exposure of the skin to the sun's ultraviolet rays, along with aging, depletes the body's natural antioxidant content that normally protects the skin. The resulting free radicals subsequently attack cellular lipids, proteins, DNA, and mitochondria, the basic building blocks of all tissues, by altering their chemical structure. But antioxidants appear to tie up the free radicals and take away their destructive power, perhaps reducing the risk of some chronic diseases.

Antioxidants slow the aging process and boost immunity by neutralizing destructive free radicals. There is revealing evidence that antioxidants help body tissue to heal quickly and prevent skin conditions. For example:

Beta-carotene: Beta-carotene is converted to vitamin A in the body. This antioxidant helps to ward off infections and is also important in vision and bone growth. Beta-carotene is found in dark-colored fruits and vegetables such as apricots, broccoli, cantaloupes, carrots, collard greens, kale, papayas, peaches, pumpkins, spinach, sweet potatoes, and tomatoes.

Selenium: This mineral helps to protect your cells against toxins and is critical to immune function. Good food sources include Brazil nuts, walnuts, cheese, eggs, enriched grain products, meats, poultry, and seafood.

Vitamin C: Scientists have long noted that vitamin C helps your skin retain collagen, giving it a more supple appearance. Vitamin C also cleans up free radicals, preventing them from damaging DNA, and helps control inflammation, aids in wound healing, and wards off infection. Try to include whole-food sources of vitamin C in your daily diet, including broccoli, cantaloupe, citrus fruits (oranges, grapefruit, tangerines), kiwifruit, peppers, potatoes, strawberries, tomatoes, and blueberries.

Vitamin E: Vitamin E is important for the maintenance of cell membranes, and many metabolic processes in the body are dependent upon healthy cell membranes — including the recuperation and growth of muscle cells. Adding almonds, lobster, corn oil, cod-liver oil, safflower oil, salmon, hazelnuts, and sunflower seeds (all rich in vitamin E) to the diet has been found effective in slowing the progression of some diseases and boosting immune response.

What About Supplements?

Studies have found *no clinical benefits* for vitamin E supplementation, as some physicians promote, for healthy skin. One study published several years ago in the *Journal of the American Medical Association* showed that supplementation with vitamin E actually increased total illness duration, with more symptoms and higher frequency of fever and activity restriction. Other findings suggest that taking high-dose vitamin E supplements (more than 400 IUs daily) actually increases mortality. For now, we suggest eating whole foods to get the benefit of this antioxidant, and talking to your doctor about your need for further supplementation.

Zinc: Zinc also has antioxidant effects and is vital to the body's resistance to infection and for tissue repair. However, high doses of zinc are toxic and may suppress immune function. It's best to ask your doctor what might be safe in your situation. Foods high in zinc include seafood, eggs, meats, whole grains, wheat germ, nuts, and seeds.

Eat More Dark Blue Foods

Dark purple fruits such as blackberries, blueberries, cranberries, cherries, and raspberries are super skin savers for sexy, ageless skin. The secret is in the color. Anthocyanins (from two Greek words meaning plant and blue) are the colorants responsible for the red, purple, and blue hues in many fruits, vegetables, and flowers. Studies show that anthocyanins play an important disease-preventive role in the body by fortifying blood vessel walls. This helps improve blood flow to the tiny blood vessels that keep eyes healthy, as well as to larger blood vessels that help maintain good circulation throughout the body. And these same foods strengthen collagen, the main component of connective tissue, which is the basis for the structure of skin.

Antioxidant Skin Savers

Skin saver fruits: Wild blueberries, cranberries, blackberries

Skin saver vegetables: Small red beans, kidney beans, and artichokes

Skin saver nuts: Pecans, walnuts, and hazelnuts

Skin saver spices: Ground cloves, ground cinnamon, and oregano

Also try: russet potatoes, black beans, plums, Gala apples, red bell peppers, pink grapefruits, onions, white grapes, corn, eggplant, cauliflower, potatoes, cabbage, leaf lettuce, bananas, apples, green beans, carrots, tomatoes, and pears

Super Berries: Blackberries, blueberries, cranberries, cherries, raspberries

Drink More Tea

Green, white, and black teas are naturally rich sources of antioxidant flavonoids (plant compounds that have beneficial actions in the human body). Some recent studies indicate that the antioxidants in tea are more powerful than those found in many fruits and vegetables, and play a role in preventing skin cancer as well as other types of cancer. Scientists have found that the intake of a single dose of tea increases total antioxidant activity in the blood. One study published in the journal *Archives of Dermatology* concluded that drinking just three glasses of oolong tea daily cut eczema symptoms for more than half of the participants in the study. Overall, green tea has the most polyphenols per cup — and polyphenols (powerful antioxidants that are responsible for the coloring in plants) have been proven to help prevent UV-induced skin cancers.

Drink Red Wine

Some new studies suggest that trans-resveratrol, a natural compound found in the skin of red grapes (and in red wine), is a powerful antioxidant — more potent than vitamin E — and conclude that it may have some chemopreventive and anti–heart disease properties.

Eat an Apple

Quercetin is one of the most abundant flavonoids in apples and demonstrates significant anti-inflammatory and antioxidant activity. Published findings from the October 2005 issue of the journal *Archives of Pharmaceutical Research* indicate that quercetin has therapeutic potential against skin aging.

Drink Your Milk

Calcium, the most abundant mineral in the body, plays a vital role in ageless skin, keeping your bones and teeth strong. But calcium must be replenished *daily* or your body will be deficient. While the calcium recommendation for adults is approximately 1,000 to 1,200 milligrams per day, the average adult gets only two-thirds to three-fourths of that amount. In fact, it is estimated that more than 80 percent of American women do not get adequate amounts of calcium in their daily diet.

Although the risk of bone fractures increases with age, new findings presented at the fifty-first annual meeting of the American College of Obstetricians and Gynecologists in May 2003 suggest that many women develop dangerously low bone mass and fractures even during the first years after menopause. The researchers said that in examinations of almost 90,000 women between the ages of

Recommended Calcium Intake

Children and Young Adults	Amount Mg/Day
6–10 years	800–1,200
11–24 years	1,200–1,500

Adult Women	Amount Mg/Day
Age 25 to menopause	1,200
After menopause	1,500
Pregnant or lactating	1,200–1,500

Consider Low-Calorie, High-Calcium Foods

If you are dieting, there are plenty of low-calorie foods that are high in calcium. Here are a few examples:

- 1 cup low-fat, calcium-fortified milk has 500 mg calcium and 80 calories
- 1 cup nonfat yogurt has 450 mg calcium and 80 calories
- 1 cup 1 percent milkfat yogurt has 450 mg calcium and 90 calories
- 1 cup low-fat milk has 300 mg calcium and 80 calories
- 1 cup fortified soy milk (set with calcium sulfate) has 300 mg calcium and 80 calories
- 1 cup fortified orange juice has 300 mg calcium and 109 calories
- 1 cup low-fat (1 percent) chocolate milk has 300 mg calcium and 110 calories
- 1 cup white beans cooked has 270 mg calcium and 250 calories
- 1 slice low-fat (2 percent) cheese has 250 mg calcium and 55 calories
- ½ cup tofu (set with calcium sulfate) has 200–400 mg calcium and 90–100 calories
- 1 cup kale (steamed) has 205 mg calcium and 30–40 calories
- 1 cup mustard greens (steamed) has 200 mg calcium and 30–40 calories
- 1 cup soybeans (cooked) has 175 mg calcium and 300 calories
- 1 cup broccoli (steamed) has 145 mg calcium and 50 calories

There are some new findings that conclude that adding calcium-rich dairy foods in a calorie-controlled diet may promote weight loss. This may give you new impetus for drinking more low-fat milk each day — stronger bones, younger-looking skin, and weight management!

fifty and sixty-four, almost one-third had bone mass low enough to put them at a higher risk of fracture.

Usually, dietary calcium can reach the recommended amounts simply by including three or four servings of calcium-rich foods each day. Low-fat dairy products (milk, cheese, and yogurt) are easy calcium sources and have an added benefit in that they contain lactose, which enhances calcium absorption. Other sources of calcium include salmon with bones, sardines, calcium-enriched juices and other food products, soy foods, and green leafy vegetables. While getting calcium from food is preferable because of the other vitamins and minerals present, you can also get your daily calcium requirement from natural dietary supplements, particularly those made from calcium carbonate or citrate. Because the body can only absorb 500 to 600 milligrams of supplemental calcium at one time, divide it into several daily doses.

Get Your Daily Vitamin D

Along with the decrease in estrogen during menopause, vitamin D production also decreases. This necessary vitamin mediates the intestinal absorption of calcium, phosphorus, magnesium, and zinc in the bone-building (and bone-loss) process. In addition, vitamin D

Food Sources of Vitamin D

Food	Vitamin D (IU)
Halibut (3 ounces)	680
Pink salmon (canned, ¼ cup)	400
Tuna (canned, ¼ cup)	130
Milk (1 cup)	100
Yoplait light yogurt (6 oz.)	80
Parkay Calcium Plus spread (1 tbs.)	60
Breakfast cereal, fortified (1 cup average)	40

is important in maintaining normal thyroid function. Some experts suggest that men and women over fifty take 800 IU of vitamin D year-round. To be sure, always talk to your doctor before adding any natural dietary supplementation or increasing the dosage of supplements you normally take.

How Much Is Enough?

It's one thing to read a food label or a magazine article — or even a book like this one — that tells you how much of any vitamin, mineral, or supplement you should be ingesting every day. It's another thing to understand what that really means and how to put it into practice. How much of all these vitamins is enough?

The Daily Value (DV) (previously called Recommended Dietary Allowance, or RDA) of a nutrient is an average daily amount that you need to consume orally to prevent a vitamin deficiency. But be forewarned: these low levels are hardly adequate for many women. Whether from deprivation diets, illness, food allergies, pregnancy, or lifestyle habits such as drinking alcohol, subtle deficiencies in vitamins and nutrients frequently occur in the body.

A new concept in the prevention of disease and the slowing of aging is "pharmacologic" dosing, or the intake of nutrients far in excess of the DV. Some anti-aging skin care authors make claims that large doses of vitamin and mineral supplements are necessary to improve health, decrease inflammation, and reverse the aging process, but the actual health benefits of supplementation are uncertain. In addition, we know that megadoses of certain vitamins and minerals have been proven harmful.

Making sense of the conflicting information regarding nutritional supplements is a difficult task, but I believe that using nutritional supplements to self-treat any medical condition or to try and reverse the changes associated with aging is risky. Also, you should always talk with your doctor or pharmacist before taking prescription medications along with nutritional supplements, to make sure there are no unwanted adverse reactions from taking both. That said, I believe that no supplement (or megasupplement) can in any way make up for poor dietary and lifestyle habits and lack of daily exercise. Eat well, be well!

Beware of Salmon-Based Diets

There's no question that fish is a good source of protein and lower in calories, fat, and cholesterol than beef or chicken. *But skin care programs that promote eating large amounts of fish or shellfish (sometimes in excess of seven times per week) to promote healthy, youthful skin have one big problem: eating that amount of fish can lead to serious health consequences.* Eating this amount of fish puts you at serious risk for having too much mercury, PCB, dioxin, and other toxic substances in your body. Sure, there are some wonderful health-boosting benefits in the omega-3 fatty acids found in salmon and many shellfish . . . but at what cost?

The risk of eating fish or shellfish tainted with mercury is of greatest concern to women of childbearing age (particularly women who are pregnant, planning to become pregnant, or nursing) and young children. Because mercury is bioaccumulative, it can be passed from the pregnant woman to the fetus and cause severe learning disabilities and other neurobehavioral disorders. Recent findings from the Centers for Disease Control (CDC) show that 8 percent of women of childbearing age in the United States have unsafe mercury levels in their bodies. This translates into more than 300,000 babies born at risk each year for impairments in language, memory, and attention span, and also delayed physical development.

But mercury is not the only toxic pollutant ingested when eating fish. Dioxins, environmental chemicals that are by-products of industrial chemicals, are readily consumed when eating the fatty tissues of fish. In fact, about 90 percent of human exposure to dioxins results from the consumption of contaminated food. In animal studies, dioxins have been found to cause nerve damage, birth defects, increased incidence of miscarriages, and significant changes in immunity. The problem is that when fish are ingested frequently over time, the dioxin builds up in the body. Again, this is especially problematic for women of childbearing age and young children, but it can have serious effects on men and women of all ages.

PCBs, once used as insulating tools in electrical transformers, are fat-soluble, persistent contaminants that accumulate in the fatty tissue of marine and other animal life. Banned in the United States in 1977, these ubiquitous pollutants are still found in our soil, lakes, rivers, and atmosphere, and are commonly found in fish and fish oil. The problem with PCB exposure is the established link with liver, skin, brain, and breast cancers. In one revealing study of 212 children born to women who had eaten Lake Michigan fish contaminated with PCBs, researchers found that children who had been exposed to PCBs prenatally — but not in the mothers' breast milk — were three times as likely to have lower average IQ scores and twice as likely to be at least two years behind in word comprehension in reading than children in the control group.

And although it was once thought that farm-raised salmon was far safer to ingest than wild salmon, groundbreaking studies have determined that a wide range of PCBs, pesticides, and other toxins are found in both farmed and wild salmon.

I believe that fish is an important part of a healthy diet, but nearly all fish — including shellfish — contains traces of mercury and other toxic chemicals. So how can you eat fish and still be healthy? I tell my clients to adhere to the recommendations of the United States Environmental Protection Agency (EPA) and the Food and Drug Administration (FDA):

1. Do not eat shark, swordfish, king mackerel, or tilefish, because they contain high levels of mercury.

2. Select fish that are lower in mercury (shrimp, canned light tuna, salmon, pollock, and catfish) and eat no more than twelve ounces (two average meals) a week of selected fish.

3. Do not eat more than six ounces of tuna per week, and if you do eat tuna, do not consume other fish during the same week. Because the popular albacore "white" tuna, has more mercury than canned light tuna, it's important to be particularly careful about your intake of this type of fish.

4. If you catch fish in local waters, eat no more than six ounces of the fish per week — and do not consume any other fish during that same week.

The EPA and FDA qualify these guidelines as being for childbearing women who may become pregnant, pregnant women, nursing mothers, and young children, but I believe all people must be cautious and consider these warnings to avoid the buildup of toxins in the body.

Fish High in Omega-3

Anchovy	Mackerel
Atlantic herring	Sardines
Atlantic salmon	Shad
Bluefish	Sturgeon
Capelin	Tuna
Dogfish	Whitefish

Phytoestrogens and Sexy, Ageless Skin

Eating just one serving of soy a day can make a dramatic difference in the health of your skin. Genistein, a component of the soybean, is classified as a phytoestrogen, or a plant component with estrogen-like effects in the body. In animal studies, researchers found a significant reduction in cancer formation in animals that drank water fortified with genistein. In dermatology trials, genistein was found to inhibit skin cancer caused by the sun's ultraviolet rays, as well as reduce photodamage (particularly UVB-induced skin burns) in humans.

In osteoporosis research, components of the soybean have been found to inhibit bone loss in animals because of the estrogen-like actions. In one Japanese study, researchers found that post-menopausal women who consumed the most soy foods, including tofu, soy milk, and soybeans, had significantly denser bones than women who consumed the least soy foods. As I've said before, strong bones are necessary to pull the skin taut and keep it from sagging.

For sexy, ageless skin, aim for one or more servings a day of soy-beans, calcium-fortified soy milk, soy cheese, or tofu. Also try the variety of soy-substitute products such as burgers, sausages, bacon, and "meat" crumbles available in the frozen-food section of your supermarket.

What About Botanical Therapies?

I have found several botanical (herbal) therapies that are helpful to some women in increasing vitality and overall energy, including the following:

Siberian Ginseng (Eleuthero)

Siberian ginseng has been used for thousands of years in traditional Chinese medicine and in Russia, and has been shown to improve energy and vitality. This botanical has been reported to increase stamina and endurance, and protect the body systems against stress-induced illness.

Horsetail

Horsetail contains the biominerals manganese, magnesium, iron, and copper necessary for the collagen and elastin biosynthesis. Horsetail also contains silicon, silica, and silicic acid, of which a portion contains elemental silicon, a vital element for healthy tissues and organs of the body including the skin, hair, nails, teeth, bones, tendons, and ligaments. Because the degradation of connective tissue is commonly associated with the aging process, silicon may also possess anti-aging properties. The high mineral content (including silicic acid) makes horsetail useful in bone and connective tissue strengthening, including preventing osteoporosis.

Red Clover

Red clover extract contains four phytoestrogen components (biochanin A, formononetin, genistein, and daidzein) that have some estrogenic activity in the body. Red clover isoflavones are primarily used for the management of menopausal symptoms and may bring some relief from hot flashes as well as help postmenopausal women maintain general health and well-being.

Ask Your Doctor Before Taking Supplements

If you decide to take herbal supplements, play it safe and talk to your doctor, pharmacist, or a certified nutritionist about side effects. Herbal therapies are not recommended for pregnant women, children, the elderly, or those with compromised immune systems. In addition, some herbs have sedative or blood-thinning qualities, which may dangerously interact with prescription medications. Others may cause gastrointestinal upset if taken in large doses.

Putting the Program into Action

Nourish for Sexy, Ageless Skin

Getting Started

If you already eat a well-balanced diet filled with foods high in antioxidants and phytochemicals, chances are you will not need to make dramatic changes in your diet to have healthy skin. However, if you have a history of deprivation dieting or eat a restricted diet, a highly processed diet, or a fast-food diet, you need to consider the nutrients necessary for tissue repair, boosting collagen, and blocking free radical damage associated with photoaging. The recommendations listed below are proven to nourish your skin and your body.

We recommend starting each day of the program with our specially formulated smoothie. In our discussions with women throughout the United States and Canada, we realized that because most were so busy juggling various responsibilities, we needed to incorporate the key nutrients for aging skin in one food. Our Super Berry Smoothie gives you the necessary nutrients for sexy, ageless skin. You can then add foods from the shopping list to create your own healing menus. Complete your daily nourishment with other foods you normally enjoy, keeping in mind the calories ingested, as

well as avoiding saturated and trans fats. It might be helpful to talk
with a registered dietitian to evaluate your dieting history and current food choices to make sure you get the essential nutrients necessary for optimal health and ageless skin.

1. Drink the Super Berry Smoothie Daily

Start each morning with a Super Berry Smoothie. Not only is the
smoothie high in the essential nutrients proven to protect and heal
skin, it will give you an eye-opening burst of protein, complex carbohydrates, the "right" fats, and phytoestrogens, along with other key
nutrients. Because our ageless-skin program is created by an experienced and trained dermatological chemist who understands formulations, we have prepared the smoothie "formula" with the precise
nutrients and amounts needed to revitalize the skin without excessive calories.

Ingredients

½ cup calcium-fortified soy milk. *Soy milk is high in phytoestrogens, calcium, magnesium, phosphorus, copper, and selenium. It is also a good source of vitamin A, vitamin B_{12}, and
manganese.*

½ cup nonfat yogurt. *Yogurt is high in protein, vitamin B_{12},
pantothenic acid, potassium, and zinc. It is a good source of
riboflavin, calcium, and phosphorus.*

1 cup fresh or frozen super berries. Use any combination of
blackberries, black raspberries, acai, wild blueberries, blueberries, raspberries, strawberries, and cherries without pits to
equal 1 cup. *Super berries are high in antioxidants as well as
folate, magnesium, potassium, copper, fiber, vitamin C, vitamin
K, and manganese.*

**½ cup chopped or crushed pineapple (in natural juice,
drained).** *Pineapple is high in vitamin C and thiamin; it also contains bromelain, a key enzyme that reduces inflammation.*

½ banana. *Bananas are high in fiber, potassium, vitamin C,
manganese, and vitamin B_6.*

1 tablespoon flax oil or freshly ground flaxseed. *Flaxseed or flax oil is a megasource for alpha linolenic acid, the plant version of omega-3 fatty acids. Flax is also high in magnesium, phosphorus, copper, thiamin, and manganese.*

2 ice cubes

Put all ingredients in a blender or food processor and process until smooth. The smoothie recipe makes two medium snack servings or one large mealtime serving.

2. Sip the Green Tea Skin Saver

While you are preparing your Super Berry Smoothie, take a few minutes to make a daily Green Tea Skin Saver. You can then keep the delicious drink in your refrigerator or take it in a thermos to work. Use this refreshing drink to quench your thirst instead of drinking high-sugar or high-caffeine drinks.

Ingredients

3 cups freshly brewed green tea. *Tea polyphenols are promising chemopreventive agents against ultraviolet-induced skin cancers.*

2 cups fresh super berries. Use any combination of wild blueberries, blackberries, raspberries, black raspberries, acai, strawberries, or cherries without pits.

1 cup pineapple juice

Club soda or ginger ale (as desired)

Brew tea; remove tea bags. Mix 3 cups of the brewed tea with the berries and pineapple juice in a large pitcher. Refrigerate until chilled. To drink, pour 1 cup of the liquid into a tall glass. Scoop up several tablespoons of the berries with the cup of liquid. Add a splash of club soda or ginger ale and enjoy the skin saver punch and the natural super fruit snacks when you would normally drink coffee, tea, or soda.

3. Keep Skin Hydrated

- Substitute coffee and tea with the Green Tea Skin Saver.
- Drink 8 glasses of mineral water daily.
- Add other super skin saver juices (alternate grape, cranberry, and pomegranate) to boost flavonols and polyphenols in your daily diet. Be sure to consider the extra calories of these juices in your daily calorie allotment.

4. Supplement Key Nutrients

An inadequate intake of several vitamins and minerals is linked to some chronic diseases, but vitamin excess is entirely possible with supplementation, particularly for fat-soluble vitamins such as vitamins A and D. Unlike other authors of skin care books, we believe that taking vitamins *does not replace* the need to nourish your body with a healthy diet. With whole foods, you get complete nutrients (known and unknown). If your diet is deficient in certain vitamins and minerals, consider the following:

- Take a generic form of "one-a-day" multivitamin.
- Be sure your multivitamin includes at least 400 micrograms per day of folic acid if you are a woman in the childbearing years.
- Add calcium supplements to meet the criteria for your age or stage, listed on page 65.
- Talk with your doctor to see if you get adequate amounts of vitamin D for boosting bone strength.
- If you are a vegetarian or vegan, getting enough vitamin B_{12} is difficult. Talk to your doctor about supplementation.
- Add essential fatty acid supplementation (marine omega-3 fatty acids or fish oil, flaxseed oil, evening primrose oil, or borage oil). Follow dosage directions on the supplement label and store supplements in a cool, dark place for safety.

5. Use the Nourish Shopping List to Plan Your Menu

When you shop for groceries, follow the perimeter of the grocery store, where the fresh foods are, and avoid the displays and inner aisles, where the packaged foods are usually stocked. Some of the foods we recommend that you keep in your kitchen include:

- **Fat-free milk, yogurt, and cheese**
- **Eggs / egg substitutes**
- **Lean beef or pork, skinless chicken, and turkey**
  - Beef: USDA Select or Choice grades of lean beef trimmed of fat, such as round, sirloin, and flank steak; tenderloin; roast (rib, chuck, rump); steak (T-bone, porterhouse, cubed); ground round
  - Pork: Lean pork, such as fresh ham; canned, cured, or boiled ham; Canadian bacon; tenderloin, center loin chop
  - Poultry: Chicken and turkey (white or dark meat, no skin)
- **Soy products, including**
  - Edamame (beans in the pod)
  - Miso (paste)
  - Meat analogs (textured soy protein)
  - Soybeans
  - Soy cheese, sour cream, cream cheese
  - Soy flour
  - Soy milk
  - Soy nuts
  - Tempeh
  - Tofu (soft; silken, firm, extrafirm)
  - Tofu (water-packed; firm or extrafirm)
- **Fish and shellfish (limit fish to two servings weekly)**
  - Anchovies
  - Atlantic herring
  - Bluefish
  - Capeline
  - Dogfish
  - Mackerel
  - Shad
  - Sardines
  - Sturgeon
  - Tuna
  - Whitefish
  - Wild salmon
- **Dried peas and beans**
  - Baked beans
  - Black beans
  - Chickpeas

- Kidney beans
- Lentils
- Navy beans
- Pinto beans
- Red lentils
- Split peas
- Soybeans
- **Fresh or frozen vegetables**
  - Artichokes
  - Asparagus
  - Beans
  - Broccoli and broccoli rabe
  - Brussels sprouts
  - Cabbage (green and purple)
  - Carrots
  - Celery
  - Cucumbers
  - Eggplant
  - Greens (kale, mustard, collard)
  - Lentils
  - Lettuce (dark green varieties)
  - Mushrooms
  - Onions
  - Peas
  - Red, orange, yellow, and green peppers
  - Spinach
  - Squash (summer and winter varieties)
  - Zucchini
- **Fresh or frozen fruits**
  - Apples
  - Apricots
  - Avocados
  - Bananas
  - Cantaloupes
  - Grapefruits
  - Honeydew melons
  - Kiwifruits
  - Lemons
  - Limes

- Mangos
- Oranges
- Papayas
- Pineapples
- Pomegranates
- Tangerines
- Tomatoes
- **Fresh or frozen super berries**
  - Blackberries
  - Acai
  - Raspberries
  - Black raspberries
  - Blueberries or wild blueberries
  - Cherries without pits
  - Strawberries
- **Juice drinks**
  - Acai
  - Pomegranate
  - Pineapple
  - Grape
  - Orange
- **Whole grains (breads, cereals, pasta)**
  - Barley
  - Bulgur
  - Bran
  - Brown rice
  - Couscous
  - Millet
  - Oats
  - Polenta
  - Quinoa
  - Whole grain bread and pasta
- **Seeds and nuts**
  - Almonds
  - Almond butter
  - Macadamia nuts
  - Peanuts
  - Pecans
  - Peanut butter

- Pumpkin seeds
- Sunflower seeds
- Walnuts
- **Green, black, and oolong tea**
- **Red and white wine**
- **Condiments and extras**
  - Extra-virgin olive oil
  - Canola oil
  - Olives (black and green)
- **Fresh or bottled herbs and spices (use instead of salt for flavoring foods)**
  - Basil
  - Bay
  - Cinnamon
  - Coriander
  - Cilantro
  - Cumin
  - Dill
  - Garlic
  - Ginger
  - Oregano
  - Paprika
  - Pepper (black, white, red pepper flakes)
  - Rosemary
  - Turmeric

6. Make Wise Food Substitutions to Nourish Your Skin

There is no secret to making wise food choices to keep your skin sexy and ageless. Review step 1 to make sure you understand the science behind the specific foods that are vital to stop photoaging and protect your skin from damaging free radicals. Then, using the following meal planner, consider the "before" and "after" food choices as you plan your daily diet.

The food selections listed below are equal in caloric value — yet the Nourish substitutions are filled with powerful nutrients that have been shown to stop photoaging and heal damaged tissue. If necessary, talk to a registered dietitian for more ways to revamp your diet and boost ageless skin.

Nourish Menu Substitutions

Normal Food Choices	Nourish Substitutions
½ cup vanilla ice milk	1 cup blueberries with ½ cup plain yogurt
Pasta with meat sauce	Whole wheat pasta with tomato/spinach sauce
Processed lunch meat on white bread	Natural peanut butter with "all fruit" blackberry jam on whole grain bread
Pepperoni pizza — white crust	Veggie pizza with broccoli, peppers, onions, and tofu cheese on a whole wheat crust
House salad with iceberg lettuce and Thousand Island dressing	Romaine and spinach salad with added almonds, pineapple, and purple onion, with olive oil vinaigrette dressing
Cinnamon raisin muffin	Zucchini/carrot/walnut muffin
Bran cereal with skim milk	Raisin bran with added super berries (blackberries, blueberries, or raspberries)
Tomato soup	Tomato soup with carrot slices and barley
Nachos and cheese	Whole grain bagel with soy cream cheese, topped with chopped dried fruits and nuts (apricots, Craisins, walnuts)
White potatoes	Sweet potatoes
Chips and onion dip	Whole wheat pita with red lentil dip
Beef chili	Vegetarian chili with black beans, kidney beans, chickpeas, and tomato chunks
Orange juice	Cranberry, pomegranate, or grape juice
White wine	Red wine
Green beans	Kale, spinach, or brussels sprouts
1 cup peach slices	1 cup blackberries, raspberries, strawberries, dark cherries, or red grapes
Hamburger and bun	Veggie burger with low-fat cheese (or soy cheese) on whole grain bun with slices of red onion, tomato, and romaine lettuce

What Does Nourish Mean to You?

The important goal of Nourish is to enhance your immune function and increase protection from photoaging and cellular changes associated with free radical damage. The scientific studies are overwhelmingly conclusive that specific nutrients in the diet can result in healthier, ageless skin. After reviewing your specific dietary needs, along with the B. Kamins, Chemist, recommendations, we know that you will eat well and look great!

Beyond Botox Recommendations for Nourish

1. Drink a Super Berry Smoothie daily.

2. Sip Green Tea Skin Saver throughout the day.

3. Keep your skin hydrated.

4. Supplement key nutrients.

5. Use the Nourish shopping list to plan your menu.

6. Make wise food substitutions for optimum nutrition.

Chapter 5

Step #2: Move

Exercise Regularly but Don't Go for the Burn

At first glance, Lena seems like the kind of woman who should have perfectly healthy, glowing skin. This thirty-eight-year-old from Dallas, Texas, is a registered dietitian (in other words, she eats right) and a marathon runner (which means she gets lots of exercise). But when Lena contacted me last year, she was in desperate search of a cure to calm her red, inflamed skin.

Lena described her skin as being "rough and irritated, with pimples on my chin and cheeks." The problem would get worse, then the symptoms would lessen — but the problem cropped up more frequently when she was training for a marathon. She tried some well-known over-the-counter topical therapies, but all of them were irritating to her skin. She even got a prescription from her dermatologist for a stronger cortisone cream to see if it would help resolve the inflammation and redness, but to no avail.

I listened to Lena talk about her lifestyle habits, particularly her long daily runs in the hot Texas sun as she trained for a marathon. I wondered whether excessive sweating (called hyperhidrosis) during her high-intensity exercise might be the cause of Lena's skin inflammation. While everyone understands the health benefits of exercise, few people realize that excessive sweating, which results when they "go for the burn," often results in irritated, inflamed skin — and even chronic acne. To have sexy, ageless skin, I suggested that Lena consider regular, moderate exercise. Let me explain why.

Excessive sweating is the secretion of sweat in amounts greater than normal, which occurs for some women during extreme exercise or as they "go for the burn." The copious amount of sweat stays on top of the skin, inducing redness, inflammation, and itching, among other skin symptoms, and can leave even the most astute health care professional puzzled as to the cause.

A certain type of sweat gland, the eccrine glands, are found over the entire body and secrete mostly water. These aren't the glands that usually produce body odor; their purpose is to allow sweat to evaporate off the skin, which lowers the body's temperature and also helps to rid the body of some waste products like salts. Many women with sensitive skin find that the dissolved salts in sweat irritate the skin, causing rashes and itching.

For women who live in warmer climates, this problem of excessive sweating may be common year-round. And it certainly makes it difficult for the ardent female athlete or those women who enjoy high-intensity exercise to have clear, attractive skin, especially during times of rigorous training.

Striking the Right Balance

So what's a health-conscious, beauty-conscious person to do? We all know the facts about exercise. Each day the media adds to the list of reasons why being active results in optimum mental and physical health. Still, almost 70 percent of women in the United States are considered sedentary, getting little or no regular exercise. This level of physical inactivity contributes to an elevated risk of coronary heart disease, hypertension, diabetes, obesity, and overall decreased quality of life. The last thing I want to do is tell Americans to exercise *less!*

The answer, in fact, isn't to exercise less — it's to exercise smarter. That's what this chapter is all about. I am passionate about exercise and activity for wellness and overall well-being. If exercise is done regularly and at a moderate intensity, any woman can enjoy the tremendous benefits of optimal health, a normal weight, and sexy, ageless skin that is not rough and irritated. Moderate exercise challenges the cardiovascular system, detoxifies the body, builds muscle and bone strength, and keeps you flexible so your joints can move in a full range of motion. Moderate exercise also increases blood flow to the skin and helps to increase cell oxygenation, nourish skin tissue, and remove toxins and cell debris.

First, I'll look briefly at a few ways exercise boosts overall health and the condition and appearance of your skin. Then I'll talk about how to combat some of the most common skin problems relating to exercise — issues such as chapped lips, blisters, rashes, and corns and calluses. Finally, I'll offer our Beyond Botox program for incorporating the right amount of exercise into your life and tips for keeping your skin healthy too.

Why Exercise Works

I don't want to belabor this point. We all know exercise is good for us, and it makes us feel good too. Let's quickly look at a few of the ways.

The Life Giver

Exercise benefits your body in many ways. Not only does it extend your life, it lets you live life more fully right now. As an example, regular exercise reduces the amount of circulating adrenaline in the body, resulting in a slower heart rate, relaxed blood vessels, and lower blood pressure.

The Body Builder

Exercise keeps muscles strong at the time in a woman's life when muscle loss naturally occurs. According to the federally funded "Women Across America" study, middle-aged women (ages forty to fifty-five) feel more aches and pains and are physically weaker than previously believed. This study confirmed that women in this age bracket often have difficulty climbing a flight of stairs, carrying groceries, and even walking around the block.

With aging, body composition changes. Even though body weight may not change, women lose muscle and gain more body fat at midlife. This age-related process, called sarcopenia, begins around age forty, when women lose about one-half pound of muscle per year, as

The Female-Athlete Triad and Problem Skin

The female-athlete triad is composed of three medical conditions that are becoming increasingly common in women athletes, specifically, eating disorders, amenorrhea (lack of menstrual periods), and osteopenia, or low bone mass. These issues are of growing concern mainly because of the media's increased pressure on teens to maintain a "perfect" body weight and be thin. Athletes in gymnastics, dancing, swimming, skating, and running are at high risk for the female-athlete triad as they strive to appear lean and fit. And these athletes are usually the ones who must deal with constantly irritated skin as a result of excess sweating.

We know that more female athletes have amenorrhea than women in the general population. Amenorrhea is associated with decreased estrogen levels, which may also be the cause of osteopenia. While low-calorie diets are usually the first predictor of eating disorders, excessive exercise, or "going for the burn," can also be a sign of an eating disorder.

Women who experience imbalanced hormones or loss of menstrual periods, exercise obsession, and low bone density at a younger age often have acne, rosacea, or other skin problems. Once one or all of the three conditions are dealt with and resolved, the skin condition usually resolves too. If you have any of these skin problems, talk to your doctor for a medical evaluation and proper treatment.

well as muscle strength and function. These finding may be disturbing, but they can be slowed and even reversed if you focus on a regular, moderate exercise program to keep body fat low and muscle mass high.

A reason to keep muscles strong: *fat burns two to three calories per pound, while muscle burns fifty calories per pound!*

The Bone Booster

There are new estimates suggesting that, along with a decrease in muscle with aging, half of all women over the age of forty-five are now affected by low bone mass, including 90 percent of women over age seventy-five. You're probably well aware of the risks of osteoporosis. This thinning of the bones and decrease in bone density greatly increases the risk of a fracture over time. Because losing bone is completely without symptoms, most of the time a woman already has osteoporosis and is not aware of it. The National Osteoporosis Foundation believes that more than 61 million Americans will have osteoporosis by 2020.

At menopause, there is a dramatic decline in estrogen, which causes rapid bone loss and can lead to devastating bone fractures. Having the strongest bones possible *before you enter menopause* is the best weapon against debilitating fractures. Regular, moderate exercise, particularly weight-bearing exercises such as walking, jogging, and dancing, can keep your bones strong.

The Skin Saver

Moderate exercise also boosts circulation and delivery of nutrients to skin cells, helping to detoxify the body and increase collagen fiber regeneration. The benefits of exercise for your skin continue after you stop moving — the relaxation you feel after exercise shows on the face, with lessened muscle tension and fewer worry lines. The skin color is also improved after exercise because of the increase in blood flow to the skin.

The Stress Reducer

Along with strengthening the body physiologically, exercise may be the easiest — and quickest — way to boost the neurotransmitter serotonin in the brain. Scientific studies show that too much stress results in low levels of serotonin, which can create aggression and feelings of anxiety or depression.

Women seem to have a greater sensitivity to changes in serotonin. For instance, mood swings following the birth of a baby, during the menstrual cycle, or with perimenopause and menopause may be triggered by the action of female hormones on neurotransmitters.

There are different ways to boost serotonin in the body, including getting more sunlight, eating certain carbohydrate foods like pasta or bagels, taking medications, and exercising. In this regard, exercise functions like a natural tranquilizer, boosting serotonin levels in the brain and also triggering the release of epinephrine and norepinephrine (chemicals that boost alertness). If you feel stressed out much of the time, exercise helps to desensitize the body to stress.

The Immune Booster

Regular, moderate exercise appears to have the advantage of jump-starting the immune system, thus helping to reduce viruses and bacteria that invade the body through the skin. One reason for this may be that exercise increases the activity of lymphocytes, called killer cells. Activity also boosts immunoglobulin in the blood, which helps combat bacteria, bacterial toxins, viruses, and other antigens capable of inflicting damage by chemically combining with cells and disrupting the body's biochemical processes.

Watch your workouts, though. A study reported in the journal *Exercise and Immunology Review* revealed that when workouts become too stressful or excessive (what we call "going for the burn"), the body produces increased amounts of the stress hormone cortisol, which can inhibit the ability of certain immune cells to work properly. In fact, some research has found that endurance athletes are at increased risk for illness during periods of prolonged training.

Keep Your Skin Healthy During Your Workout

You know that exercise is beneficial for overall health, but being active and moving around daily is particularly valuable for your skin, to keep it nourished and healthy. I already told you the skin care risks of pushing yourself too hard and going for the burn. Instead, I recommend exercising regularly and moderately to take advantage of the incredible healing aspects of physical activity without excessive irritants (sweat) damaging the skin.

No matter what type of exercise you do, the chances are great that you will experience some sort of skin problem as a result —

Are Sunless Tanning Lotions Safe?

Many women enjoy looking tan but do not want to damage their skin with the sun's ultraviolet rays. Sunless tanning lotions give a golden "sun-kissed" look without causing photodamage. That's a great thing, and if these products promote less exposed time in the sun, it sounds like a wonderful solution to sun-damaged skin . . . right?

Not necessarily. Users of these "tans in a bottle" must remember to use a daily application of sunscreen in addition to their tanning lotion. They don't always do so, and the tanning product itself does not protect you from harmful UV rays.

I find some cause for concern in the products themselves, as well. The main ingredient in the sunless tanning products is dihydroxyacetone (DHA), which combines with amino acids in the skin to form brown compounds called melaninoids. Uneven application of such a product will produce streaked skin coloring. To maintain this type of tan, the self-tanning product has to be applied frequently, and the long-term effects of these products haven't been studied. To date, sunless tanning lotions have not been banned by the FDA, but in my opinion, there are better and safer ways to have healthy, beautiful skin!

effects such as blisters, sunburn, and painful corns and calluses. Take a look at the following pages so you won't leave your skin at risk for infection or even permanent tissue damage.

Acne

Problem: Ill-fitting equipment such as a bike helmet, knee or elbow pads, and even sports clothing made from nylon can rub on the skin during exercise and cause redness, irritation, and acne.

Skin Saver: Exercise-related acne is usually caused by friction or something that touches the skin (sweat, chemicals, clothing), rather than something wrong internally. Avoid activities where fabrics or equipment can rub or irritate the skin. For instance, some women find that the weight equipment at a gym increases rubbing and sweat on the skin, resulting in bumps, rashes, and pimples. Women who wear helmets while cycling often have a band of irritated skin where the helmet touches their face. Some find that wearing a soft knit hat under the helmet keeps it from rubbing directly on the skin. Some of this is unavoidable, but if you are extremely sensitive, select a moderate-intensity exercise that does not require equipment or special clothing that has prolonged contact with your skin.

Blisters

Problem: Most women have experienced blisters with exercise, whether from a poorly fitted shoe rubbing on tender skin, an allergy, a fungal infection, or from a sunburn. The fluid inside a blister is leaked from blood vessels in underlying skin layers after minor damage (such as your shoe rubbing on your heel).

Skin Saver: The best way to treat a blister is to protect it from tearing by covering it loosely with a gauze bandage. If you accidentally tear the blister, causing its liquid to secrete, be sure to keep it clean and loosely covered with a gauze bandage. You don't want the top of the gauze to stick to the skin, nor do you want dirt or bacteria to enter the blister. If the blister becomes red, expands in size, or releases any discharge other than clear liquid, call your doctor.

It's also important to always wear shoes that are comfortable and provide good support when you exercise. Inappropriate shoes increase the risk of blisters and calluses. Studies show that most women wear their shoes too small, which can greatly increase pressure on the feet and ankles, resulting in damage to the skin. Get shoes that support your weight yet don't put abnormal pressure on the skin or joints.

To find the best-fitting shoe, talk to a podiatrist (foot doctor) or go to a specialty shoe store. The doctor may prescribe orthotics or a specially designed insert for your shoe that helps to alleviate heel or ankle pain or abnormal rubbing on the skin.

Corns and Calluses

Problem: Corns and calluses are extremely common problems, especially with age. Not only are these thickenings on the hands or feet unsightly, but they can cause great pain. When there is repeated pressure or friction on the skin, a thickening or callus will form on the stratum corneum (the outermost layer of skin). Repeated pressure or rubbing can also cause a corn.

Skin Saver: Avoiding poorly fitting shoes is the best way to reduce the chance of a corn or callus. To remove a corn or callus, carefully shave the excess tissue with a clean implement. Use an emery board or file, or a commercial corn or callus remover in liquid or plaster form. If you find no relief from these self-help tips, or the corn or callus is extremely painful or large, check with your primary care doctor or a podiatrist (foot doctor). There are easy ways to treat or remove a corn or callus in a medical setting that can provide you with quick relief.

Chapped Lips

Problem: Chapped lips are a common problem for women who exercise regularly, especially during the dry winter months. Chapped lips are usually caused by environmental factors, such as extreme cold or excessive heat, wind, and low water content in the air. Compulsive lip wetting and some medications can accelerate lip dehydration.

Skin Saver: Choose a lip balm that contains petrolatum, castor oil, paraffin, squalane, carnauba wax, zinc oxide, octinoxate, benzophenone-3, or Bio-Maple compound.

Cracked Lips

Problem: Another common problem with exercise during the winter months is cracking of the corners of the lips (called perleche).

Skin Saver: Apply zinc oxide to the corners of the mouth. Zinc seals in moisture and acts as an anti-inflammatory and anti-yeast agent.

Cuts and Scratches

Problem: Whether from falling down on a rocky path during a morning hike, getting scraped on exercise equipment, or bumping into the biker in front of you while doing a mountain ride, exercise increases the chance of cutting or scratching the skin. The problem is that once the skin is broken, bacteria can enter the wound, causing infection.

Skin Saver: Apply first aid immediately upon injuring the skin. If the wound or scratch is bleeding, cover it with a clean cloth and apply pressure for two or three minutes until the bleeding stops. If the wound is not gaping or bleeding much, apply an antiseptic such as Betadine spray and cover the wound with a gauze bandage. Try to avoid letting the gauze stick to the wound. After three to four days of healing, apply an antibiotic ointment to the wound and rub it gently over the scab. Look for ointments containing antibiotics such as polymyxin B and bacitracin.

Most cuts and scrapes heal quickly with regular cleaning and covering. For a deep wound, seek medical help.

Environmental Chemicals

Problem: Many environmental pollutants can trigger skin problems for those who exercise a lot out of doors. For instance, avoid running in polluted industrial areas or exercising in outdoor areas that have been recently sprayed with weed killers. Chlorine in the swimming pool is another exercise hazard for both the skin and the hair.

Skin Saver: Shower immediately after exercising or swimming in a chlorinated pool. Leave skin wet and generously apply a moisturizing body lotion containing ingredients such as Bio-Maple, glycerin, urea, or sodium lactate to counteract the drying effect of the chlorine. While the face is wet, immediately apply an appropriate face cream or lotion that contains petrolatum, squalane, sodium PCA, or hyaluronic acid.

Rashes

Problem: Many women complain of skin rashes after exercise, especially if their thighs rub together or clothing irritates the skin. This bright red patch is nothing more than inflamed skin, or dermatitis. Sometimes a rash occurs when you trap wetness next to the skin exercising in hot, humid conditions. The warm, moist area provides the perfect environment for microbes to grow, resulting in an irritation rash or a yeast rash. Yeast rashes that are normally found on the skin can take over and grow out of control, leaving the skin reddish, puffy, and slightly warm to the touch.

Skin Saver: The best way to avoid dealing with rashes is to take precautions ahead of time. For instance, remove sweaty clothing immediately after exercise, and then rinse the sweat and bacteria off your skin with a cool shower. Get out of a wet bathing suit immediately to avoid a yeast infection or an itchy rash.

If you do get a rash, try a cream that contains zinc oxide, bisabolol, allantoin, or petrolatum to help protect the skin and promote healing. These products should be gently applied directly on clean skin to help it heal. Also, avoid the use of powders and cornstarch, as these stick to the skin, forming the perfect breeding ground for bacteria.

Sunburn

Problem: Prevention of sun damage altogether is our utmost recommendation for sexy, ageless skin. Nonetheless, we realize that avoiding the sun's ultraviolet rays is not always possible.

Skin Saver: If you do get a mild sunburn, it is important to take healing measures immediately.

Even though over-the-counter products containing topical anesthetics such as benzocaine are touted as being effective for sunburn, there is little scientific evidence on their effectiveness. To treat the painful symptoms, use cold compresses, nonsteroidal anti-inflammatory drugs (NSAIDs) or acetaminophen, antihistamines, and low-potency topical corticosteroids.

Moisturize to limit inflammation and peeling. Even if you have a sunburn, continue to follow sun-preventive strategies by wearing sunscreen daily, avoiding UV exposure, and wearing wide-brimmed hats, sunglasses, and loose-fitting clothes with long sleeves and long pants.

Get with the Beat!

Researchers in the Department of Physical Therapy at Springfield College in Massachusetts found that people who exercise to music stay with it longer than if they work out in silence. Men and women riding stationary bikes rode from 25 to 29 percent longer listening to their favorite tunes.

Hygiene Tip

Always shower immediately after exercising to rinse sweat off the skin. If sweat is left on the skin, bacteria can grow and trigger outbreaks of pimples or acne.

Putting the Program into Action

Move for Sexy, Ageless Skin

1. See Your Health Care Provider Before Starting This Step

If you are over fifty and have not been active for while, talk to your physician or health care provider before you begin exercising.

2. Set Personal Goals

Write down on paper the reasons you are starting a regular, moderate exercise program. For example, are you trying to get in shape? Lose weight? Build muscle? Improve mood? Or are you exercising because of the overall health benefits to the body and mind? No matter what your reason, putting it down in writing will help you stay focused on why you are setting aside time for this, especially when life's interruptions test your dedication.

3. Exercise Regularly at Least Thirty Minutes a Day, Five Days a Week

To meet your exercise requirement, it is important to select those activities you really enjoy or you will drop out of the program within weeks. Keep in mind that "exercise" does not always have to mean going to a fitness center or walking on a treadmill. Exercise can also be those household or daily activities you enjoy doing or must do, such as gardening, mowing the lawn, washing windows, sweeping, and carrying in bags of groceries. Playing with children or grandchildren is yet another healthy way to move around more and fulfill your moderate-exercise requirements.

While the studies are inconclusive, it is thought that spending five to ten minutes before and after exercise stretching, walking in place, or doing calisthenics is helpful in warming up and cooling down the body. Stretching should be a slow and dynamic movement, with the stretch held for thirty seconds. Do not bounce into the stretch or during the stretch.

Choose from These Moderate Exercises and Daily Activities

Moderate Exercise	Daily Activities
Aerobics (low-impact)	Bending while cleaning or gardening
Ballroom dancing	Climbing stairs
Biking	Cutting the grass
Golf (carrying the clubs)	Dusting
Hiking	Gardening
Mall-walking	Housekeeping
Stair-climbing	Lifting packages or children
Swimming	Raking leaves
Walking	Walking to store, work, friend's home
Water aerobics	Washing windows

4. Add Resistance Training Two to Three Times a Week

Strengthening exercises help to build the strong muscles and tendons needed to support the joints in the body. You can use resistance equipment or even your own body as resistance to build muscle strength in your arms, shoulders, chest, trunk, back, hips, and legs.

For your strengthening workout, start with a weight that you can easily lift ten times, with the last two repetitions being increasingly difficult. A weight that becomes difficult at eight repetitions has been shown in studies to be an effective stimulus for strengthening and toning muscles. Some women start at one to two pounds; others start at fifteen to twenty pounds. Find the right weight for you. As you gain in strength, you can increase the weight in one- or two-pound increments.

Do each lift slowly to get maximum benefit. Aim for ten minutes two to three times a week. Studies show that you only need to do one set of the exercise to derive benefit. Doing more sets might fatigue the muscles or defeat your purpose of moderate training. Some good choices for moderate resistance training include:

- Isometric rope
- Elastic bands
- Swim gloves and kickboard, using the water as resistance
- Free weights
- Resistance machines

5. Add Flexibility Exercises

Range-of-motion, or flexibility, exercises involve moving a joint as far as it will go (without pain) or through its full range of motion. When done correctly, stretching the body and moving your joints through their full range of motion feels good and helps increase blood flow throughout the body. Increased blood circulation helps to boost skin health.

Your stretching routine should be very specific and include all the major muscle groups, including the shoulders, hips, pelvis, buttocks, thighs, and calves. Carefully move to the maximum range of motion of the joint that you are able to do easily, without pain or unusual discomfort. Then slightly increase the motion until you feel resistance or discomfort. Do this only one time. Ask your doctor, physical therapist, or personal trainer for a complete list of stretching and range-of-motion exercises.

6. Incorporate Mini Workouts When You Are Busy

If you have no time to commit to exercise, we recommend trying to get it in three or four ten-minute segments. Consider the following:

10-minute run on a treadmill before work

10-minute bike ride before work

10-minute walk around the parking lot before entering the
building

10-minute walk on a treadmill midday

10-minute swim in your pool

10-minute low-impact aerobics routine

10-minute tai chi video session

10-minute stretching exercises

10 minutes of walking in place (1,000 steps equals half a mile)

7. Use Skin-Saving Strategies When Exercising

- Always wear sunscreen.
- Wear light-colored, loose fitting clothing. Dark fabrics increase your body temperature and reduce evaporation, causing sweat to remain on the skin. Loose-fitting clothing allows air to pass over your skin, providing for sweat evaporation and cooling.
- Exercise when it's cool and avoid the midday sun.
- Wear a light-colored hat to protect your skin from the sun's rays.

Beyond Botox Recommendations for Move

1. See your health care provider for a checkup to get a go to exercise.

2. Set personal goals.

3. Exercise regularly at least thirty to forty-five minutes a day, five days a week.

4. Add resistance training two to three times a week.

5. Add flexibility exercises.

6. Incorporate mini workouts on days you are too busy to exercise.

7. Use skin-saving strategies when you exercise.

Chapter 6

Step #3: Rest

Get Quality Sleep to Rejuvenate Skin

Carole, a forty-three-year-old registered nurse from a small town near Des Moines, Iowa, wrote to me seeking guidance on how to treat the dramatic skin changes she was undergoing during perimenopause. Working full-time on the geriatric ward of a large county hospital, Carole often pulled twelve-hour shifts to have more days off each month to spend with her two children. While she loved nursing, Carole admitted that the extended shifts were hard on her marriage and really sapped her energy. Lately, her husband and friends had commented that she was looking more wan and tired. The dark circles under her eyes never seemed to go away, no matter how much concealer she applied each morning. And the small wrinkles around her eyes and mouth were rapidly becoming more pronounced.

Carole thought maybe a change to her skin care routine was in order. But after talking a bit with her, I realized that there were other lifestyle changes that Carole needed to address first — and getting more, better rest was at the top of the list.

The Price Your Skin Pays for Losing Sleep

Along with changing your diet and exercising moderately each day, an essential strategy for sexy, ageless skin is getting enough healing sleep. Over the past decade, we have learned much about the consequences of sleep deprivation. Through numerous scientific studies, sleep experts now conclude that if you cheat on your sleep, you can almost count on premature skin aging. In a revealing study reported in the *Journal of Investigative Dermatology*, researchers tested sleep-deprived women and found that a lack of sleep left their skin more susceptible to outside allergens and bacteria. Other studies have reported a decrease in growth hormone with sleep restriction, resulting in thinner, dryer skin and even hair loss.

Although you cannot erase the sleep deprivation of years past, you can start now to evaluate your sleep habits and change those over which you have control. That's why all women should understand the characteristics of normal sleep and how any deviation from this norm may result in illness and unhealthy, fragile skin that looks old years before it should. Take my client Amy as an example.

A senior sales representative with a large software company in the Northeast, forty-nine-year-old Amy thrived on her fast-paced lifestyle and corporate contacts. A single mother of two young adults, Amy resided in Boston and flew to large cities throughout New England and Canada each week, meeting with executives and their sales teams and attending cocktail parties and late-night formal dinners.

Amy wrote to me in hopes of finding "a miracle lotion or cream" that would revitalize her drab, blotchy complexion. Within her letter was a wealth of pertinent information as to why Amy's skin looked much older than her actual age:

> While I sleep well on the weekends, averaging about seven to eight hours each night, on weeknights, I can forget sleep altogether. My mind is on red alert, thinking of all the business decisions I must make, early-bird flights I have to catch, new clients I must call, and how my kids are surviving so far away from me at college. With my mind in high gear, I end up tossing and turning all night long. After about four hours of broken sleep, I awaken the next morning feeling achy, exhausted, and irritable — and then I have to get dressed, meet clients for coffee, and be sharp to make deals. Not only am I sleep deprived, but after the nights I cannot sleep, I look years older than my actual age. My skin is noticeably thinner and transparent, and I cannot find any

makeup or concealer that effectively masks the dark under-eye circles and skin blotches.

Most women who are juggling work, family, and the accompanying stress can relate to Amy's feelings of being on red alert, especially when you add the declining hormones associated with perimenopause and menopause. Findings indicate that millions of women Amy's age suffer from disordered sleep, especially insomnia, which is characterized by difficulty falling asleep or maintaining sleep, or an inability to feel rested despite adequate time spent in bed. With age, the prevalence of insomnia increases as sleep time decreases, even though the time spent in bed might increase.

And, as Amy has also experienced, at midlife the onset to sleep is lengthened, making it more difficult to fall asleep even though nighttime awakenings are more frequent, which leads to restlessness and poor-quality sleep. Sleep problems are also commonly associated with acute (short-term) and chronic (long-term) stress, as stress hormones such as cortisol pour through the body, putting the nervous system on high alert. Is it any wonder that Americans spent $2.1 billion on prescription sleep aids last year and bought more than 600 million over-the-counter sleep tablets?

Getting inadequate sleep for a few nights probably won't cause you harm. If you continue to get poor sleep for weeks on end, however, the immune system weakens and there is increased risk of chronic illness such as heart disease, obesity, diabetes, and cancer, including melanoma and other types of serious skin cancers. Moreover, sleep deprivation is cumulative — it adds up. For instance, although Amy said she needed eight hours of sleep each night, she actually got about four hours of sleep a night for four nights each week. Amy missed a total of sixteen hours of sleep each week. This serious sleep debt is equivalent to two full nights each week without sleep and results in severe sleep deprivation. Over time, Amy will pay the price for this sleep debt in weakened immune function and in premature skin aging.

I know it's not easy to get adequate sleep each night, especially when you're out late with clients or up several times a night with young children. In this chapter I will talk about some reasons sleep becomes increasingly difficult with age, particularly for women during perimenopause and menopause. I'll look briefly at how hormones influence sleep and at the normal stages of sleep that are necessary for optimum health. Then I'll talk about how sleep influences your skin by affecting your immunity, your weight, and even the levels of human growth hormone, which is necessary to feeling energetic and youthful, in the body. Next I'll assess skin problems that accompany poor sleep, such as dark under-eye circles, flaky skin, and increased lines and wrinkles. Finally, I'll give you our Beyond Botox program for regulating your sleep as you establish your personal "sleep zone" and learn some quick ways to calm your mind and body before crawling into bed each night.

Insomnia Alert

According to the National Institute on Aging, one out of eight individuals in their twenties has chronic insomnia, and one out of five people ages fifty to sixty-four and one in four people over age sixty-five experience this sleep disorder.

Can't Sleep? Blame Your Hormones

Many sleep experts are beginning to define the function that hormone levels have in determining the quality and quantity of sleep. Not only does lack of sleep cause you to look old and tired, women are more prone than men to have difficulty maintaining quality sleep.

Menstruation. Stages and conditions in the female life cycle such as menstruation, pregnancy, perimenopause, and menopause have a direct relationship to a woman's fluctuating hormones. The changing levels of the hormones estrogen and progesterone throughout these times cause women to sleep well or barely sleep at all. For example, comprehensive studies demonstrate that women have more sleep disruptions — including difficulty getting to sleep, awakenings, sleep disturbances, and vivid dreams — during the *premenstrual* and *menstrual* time than the rest of the month. Although the hormone estrogen increases rapid eye movement (REM) sleep, the deep stage of sleep when dreams occur, progesterone, which rises midcycle after ovulation, causes feelings of fatigue or drowsiness. When menstruation begins and progesterone levels fall, women usually have difficulty falling asleep and often experience the lowest quality of sleep for a few days. As the woman's cycle begins again, normal sleep (which is not always good sleep) usually returns.

Childbirth. Pregnancy, childbirth, postpartum recovery, and breastfeeding create physical and emotional stress that disrupts sleep. Not only are hormones imbalanced in pregnancy, with a surge of sleep-inducing progesterone, the growing uterus applies pressure on the bladder, making nighttime an active time for most moms. Sleep variations during pregnancy usually occur during the first and third trimesters.

During the postpartum period, or the six to eight weeks following delivery, sleep is still difficult for many women, as the imbalanced hormones and the newborn's cries keep moms on high alert. For women who are breastfeeding, nursing a baby on demand for months can also result in a huge sleep debt.

Perimenopause and menopause. In perimenopause, hormone fluctuations again are blamed for disturbed sleep. Many women report difficulty in falling asleep, difficulty staying asleep, and fatigue and fogginess upon arising. At this stage in the life cycle, many women experience hot flashes and attribute their sleep arousals to increased body temperature and night sweats. Some women report that hot flashes occur for several months; in others, these disruptions last for ten years or longer, if they start at the beginning of perimenopause. Adding to these stresses, at this life stage many women are juggling raising teenagers, managing careers, and caring for aging parents — all of which can increase anxiety, resulting in feelings of overload and poor sleep.

According to the National Institutes of Health, the prevalence of sleep disturbance in women varies from 16 to 42 percent in premenopause, from 39 to 47 percent in perimenopause, and from 35 to 60 percent in postmenopause. While there are no easy answers for resolving sleep deprivation, with more women avoiding hormone replacement therapy, we need immediate answers and specific targeted therapies to resolve these problems.

Sleep 101

It may seem as if all sleep is the same throughout the night. However, there are very specific stages of sleep, and each one serves a unique function. For instance, when you first fall asleep, you immediately move from a light sleep to a deeper stage of sleep. It is during this deep-sleep state that you experience metabolic and tissue restoration. Human growth hormone is secreted, and stress hormones such as cortisol are at a minimum.

As we age, medical problems, medications, and daytime naps, along with fluctuating hormones, often interfere with restful sleep, resulting in shorter periods of deep sleep and increased daytime fatigue or sleepiness. In addition, poor sleep affects every part of your life — including your looks, resulting in pasty, dry skin, transparent skin, increased wrinkling, discoloration, and dark under-eye circles. Before we look at how to solve these common skin ailments, let's take a moment to explore the various stages of sleep to give you a better understanding of the impact sleep has on the skin and motivate you to make some nighttime changes.

The Stages of Sleep

Some think of sleep as "down time," but it is really an active state as complex as wakefulness. The brain is not resting during sleep but rather involved in a wide variety of activities. Your sleep quality is measured by the amount of delta sleep you get. This deepest level of sleep occurs mostly during the first third of the night. Growth hormone secretion is highest during delta sleep, and some researchers believe that this stage is most important for growth and repair of body tissue.

Stage 1 sleep is the transition from wakefulness to deeper sleep. This is the lightest stage of sleep.

Stage 2 sleep, sometimes called intermediate sleep, typically accounts for 40 to 50 percent of total sleep time.

Stages 3 and 4 sleep, also called delta sleep, are frequently referred to as deep sleep, or slow-wave sleep. These stages account for 20 percent of total sleep time in young adults.

Both the quantity and quality of sleep change significantly with aging. Usually, deep sleep (stages 3 and 4, or delta) declines with age, and light sleep (stage 1) increases. The number of arousals and the amount of wakefulness also increase in later years. Not surprisingly, young children have particularly large proportions of delta sleep, which increases if they are sleep deprived or very tired. This explains why trying to wake a young child may be difficult. Environmental noise during the nighttime hours usually arouses older adults because of the smaller proportion of delta sleep.

8 Sexy, Ageless Skin Sleep Benefits

1. Conserves energy
2. Prevents fatigue
3. Provides organ respite
4. Relieves tension
5. Boosts immune function
6. Triggers the release of human growth hormone
7. Controls appetite
8. Normalizes weight

How Sleep Affects Your Skin

Today, adults of all ages suffer with chronic sleep loss as a common response to the pressures of modern society, whether staying up too late or awakening too early to accomplish tasks. In fact, over the past forty years, the proportion of adults in the United States sleeping less than seven hours per night has increased from 16 to 37 percent.

The problem is that even occasional sleep problems make daily life feel more stressful and less productive because the body and mind need consistent, restful sleep to function optimally. Let's look at how sleep — or lack thereof — affects your immunity, your overall health, and your weight . . . factors that can affect your quest for sexy, ageless skin.

Sleep Regulates Immunity

Skin is a natural defense mechanism against the outside world and plays a big role in regulating your immune system. As discussed, a weakened immune system can result in ailments such as frequent colds, sore throats, allergies, skin problems, and even skin cancer.

From scientific studies, we know that exposure to viruses and bacteria usually results in no health problems *if* your immune system is strong. Yet when faced with sleep deprivation, the immune system cannot work at full capacity. When your immune system malfunctions, it yields to autoimmune diseases such as some types of arthritis, allergy, or asthma. When the immune system is depleted, bacteria, viruses, or toxins can overwhelm the body and possibly result in cancer or other life-threatening diseases. Studies have shown that sleep deprivation ultimately reduces immunity and results in skin that is dehydrated, wrinkled, pale, and less able to repair itself quickly.

Sleep Helps with Weight Management

If the connection between sleep problems and aging skin isn't troublesome enough, there is substantial evidence from numerous sleep studies indicating that sleeping less has negative metabolic consequences and may be the cause of weight gain. Dr. Eve Van Cauter and her colleagues at the University of Chicago demonstrated this in findings published in the *Annals of Internal Medicine* (2004). In the study, healthy young men underwent two days of sleep restriction (four hours a night) and then two days of sleep extension (ten hours per night) six weeks later. During this time, researchers monitored their calorie intake and physical activity. Researchers found that sleep restriction was associated with increased hunger and appetite (in particular for calorie-dense foods with high carbohydrate content). The volunteers who slept only four hours a night for two nights had an 18 percent decrease in leptin, a hormone that signals to the brain that there is no need for more food, and a 28 percent increase in ghrelin, a hormone that triggers hunger, increases food intake, and produces weight gain. In other words, losing sleep makes you crave high-calorie, high-carb foods and disrupts your body's ability to know it's had enough.

Sleep Boosts Human Growth Hormone

Human growth hormone (HGH), secreted by the pituitary gland of the brain, declines as we age. A microscopic protein substance, HGH is secreted in short pulses during deep sleep and after exercise. The decline of growth hormone with age is directly associated with cardiovascular disease, increased body fat, osteoporosis, gray hair, wrinkles, decreased energy, reduced sexual function, and other symptoms. Many of these symptoms are found in younger adults who have growth hormone deficiencies. Increasing deep sleep to promote an increase in HGH might help delay many of the conditions we associate with aging.

Psychological Consequences of Sleep Deprivation

Mood swings
Irritability
Depression, distrust, and paranoia
Lack of patience
Intolerance
Cognitive dysfunction
Memory loss
Difficulty learning
Decreased attention span
Negligence
Reduced performance

Keep Your Sleep Healthy for Beautiful Skin

Even when you try diligently to prepare for restful sleep, there will be nights when you toss and turn, especially when you are out late or feeling stressed. After a night with little sleep, the most common effects on the skin are spots, rashes, flakiness, and added fine lines or deep wrinkles. Let's look at some of the most common skin problems associated with lack of sleep and some quick and easy ways to resolve them.

Pillow Creases in Skin

Problem: Morning lines after sleeping on a pillow.

Skin Saver: Try to change your sleep position when you first crawl into bed each night. For instance, if you normally sleep with your face buried in the pillow, try a new position, such as sleeping on your back, and elevate your head by sleeping on two pillows instead of one. Sleeping in the same position every night often leaves permanent lines on the skin.

Dull, Dry Skin

Problem: Lack of sleep that results in dull, dry skin, making you look older than you really are.

Skin Saver: Soak and slather when skin is tired and dry looking. Soak in a warm bath or shower, and then immediately supersaturate the skin with a moisturizer to revitalize it and keep it looking soft and supple.

Morning Puffiness

Problem: Skin puffiness upon awakening. Morning puffiness is the result of water accumulating in the tissues during the night. This condition is worsened by salt, alcohol, and little sleep. Allergies and sunburn can also increase the chance of morning puffiness.

Skin Saver: Sleep with your head elevated on two pillows at night if you are prone to morning puffiness. Change your diet to avoid salty foods and alcohol. If you have allergies, talk to your doctor about one of the newer nonsedating antihistamines, such as Claritin, that might help under-eye puffiness.

Under-eye Pouches

Problem: Under-eye pouches and swelling.

Skin Saver: Fluids redistribute while you snooze and can collect around the eyes. Sleep with your head on two pillows to allow fluids to drain if your neck condition permits. In addition, applying a cold compress (or a bag of frozen vegetables) for five minutes to reduce swelling. Cold packs reduce inflammation by constricting blood vessels. Follow with a firming eye treatment that contains antioxidants, physiological humectants, hydrating agents, ceramides (phospholipids and spingolipids), and hyaluronic acid.

For some women this puffiness can become more permanent over time. As membranes in the eyelid weaken, the small fat pads located below the eye begin to move forward, forming bulges or "bags" that just don't go away. Unfortunately, these bags tend to be genetically controlled and can only be alleviated by surgically removing or repositioning them.

Dark Circles

Problem: Dark blue or purple under-eye circles. With age, the skin under the eye becomes thinner and more transparent. When you are stressed and sleep deprived, this eye area skin looks especially fragile and thin. There is a genetic predisposition to dark under-eye circles, and they can become more prominent with age as the skin becomes translucent, with purple or blue blood vessels showing through. Crow's-feet and fine lines can also develop during this period, accentuating the problem.

Skin Saver: Aim for seven to eight hours of sleep each night to ensure you are well rested. If your circles are the result of allergies, talk to your doctor about an antihistamine that does not cause drowsiness. Also, use under-eye concealer during the day.

Large Open Pores

Problem: Large open pores after a late-night party.

Skin Saver: Your pores may appear larger and open when you stay up late and drink alcohol. Although you cannot change the size of your pores, there are ways to make them appear smaller with an astringent toner that contains zinc sulfate or alum. Also try a clay mask that contains bentonite and exfoliate with a product that contains glycolic acid. For oily skin, use a mild cleanser to remove excess shiny sebum.

Putting the Program into Action

Rest for Sexy, Ageless Skin

Our sleep needs vary, and achieving your personal sleep balance is the key to active aging. Using the many strategies in this section, you can begin to resolve some of your sleep issues. Over time, increased sleep will result in healthier skin and a more glowing, youthful appearance.

1. Find Your Sexy, Ageless Skin Sleep Zone

Here's something your doctor may not tell you: not every woman needs eight hours of sleep a night to have sexy, ageless skin. Studies continue to confirm that getting seven to eight hours of sleep each night is consistent with optimal health, but there are those individuals who thrive on six hours a night and look great. These people have no health complaints and function well on what might seem like inadequate sleep to others. (But it's important to note that individuals who sleep fewer than four or more than ten hours have been reported to have increased rates of mortality.)

It is important for you to find your own sexy, ageless skin sleep zone. No one can dictate how much sleep is best for you — except you. Start by keeping a daily sleep log, using the chart on page 110. Beginning with Monday, write down the amount of sleep you got on Sunday night. Then each consecutive day of the week, jot down the amount of sleep you got the previous night. Also, write down your feelings upon awakening and then again throughout the day. Were you alert and energetic? Did your eyes look bright and rested? Or were you moody and inattentive? Did your skin look pasty or puffy?

We have done the first chart, Keri's, as a sample. You can see how seven to seven and a half hours of sleep may be ideal for Keri after reviewing the chart. Now copy the sample seven-day chart (page 110) to create your own sleep log. (You'll need three copies of the chart for this step.) Fill in the appropriate blanks of this chart each day for three weeks, addressing each category. Once you have filled in the blanks for three weeks, review the chart and your responses. You should get a good idea of the optimum sleep amount for you — the amount necessary each night for you to feel great, be active, and have sexy, ageless skin.

Keri's Sleep Zone Chart

Day of the Week	Hours of Sleep	Mood Upon Awakening	Alertness the Next Day	Skin Tone the Next Day	Mood the Entire Day
Monday	6	Irritable	Needed two cups of coffee to function	Swollen under-eye circles	Improved with time
Tuesday	7	Good	Completed many projects	Healthy	Even mood
Wednesday	7.5	Good	Highly productive	Healthy	Positive mood
Thursday	6.5	Irritable	Felt fatigued all day	Under-eye circles were dark purple/ blue	Sluggish and low mood
Friday	9	Irritable	Felt sluggish all day	Had wrinkles from sleeping hard on pillow	Took a nap
Saturday	7	Great!	High energy	Healthy	Got two new clients!
Sunday	7.5	Good	Productive	Healthy	Enjoyed my day

2. Prepare Your Mind and Body for Sleep

Once you have established your sleep zone, use the following suggestions to prepare your body and mind for rest and to create an atmosphere conducive for sound sleep.

Sleep only as much as needed to feel refreshed and healthy the following day, not more. Always awaken at the same time, even if you go to bed late. On weekends, continue to awaken at the same time. If you must nap, make sure it's for no longer than twenty to thirty minutes. In a study published in March 2004 in the journal *Psychosomatic Medicine,* Dr. Daniel Kripke of the University of California, San Diego, found that those who sleep longer than eight hours

Your Sleep Zone Chart

Day of the Week	Hours of Sleep	Mood Upon Awakening	Alertness the Next Day	Skin Tone the Next Day	Mood the Entire Day
Monday					
Tuesday					
Wednesday					
Thursday					
Friday					
Saturday					
Sunday					

a night and those who sleep fewer than seven hours a night report more sleep complaints than people who sleep seven to eight hours. Find your sleep zone and then be consistent in getting the amount of sleep you need.

Avoid salty foods. Following a reduced-sodium diet helps some insomniacs sleep more soundly. Avoid chips, crackers, nuts, and other foods high in sodium before bedtime.

Avoid exercise and intense mental activities four hours before bedtime. Moderate daily exercise, as explained in step 2 of the Beyond Botox program, will help to deepen sleep as it reduces stress and lengthens slow-wave (delta) sleep. But exercise before bedtime can increase alertness and make it difficult to rest. Also, stay off the computer and put away work-related tasks several hours before bed so your mind has time to wind down.

Make sure your bedroom is suited for sleep. Wear earplugs if you are bothered by noises while sleeping. Some people find that white noise — a machine that produces a humming sound or tuning the radio to a station that has gone off the air — helps. Also, get black-out shades for your room so it is fully dark. Light is a cue for the body to awaken; darkness signals relaxation and sleep. Wear a sleep mask if you are ultrasensitive to light and find it disrupts your sleep time. Turn your clock's face to the wall so you are not tempted to check the time all night long.

Before bedtime, have a light high-carb snack (bread, cereal, or pasta). Serotonin is a mood-elevating brain chemical that often has a calming effect and can result in sounder sleep. Eating foods high in complex carbohydrates can raise levels of serotonin in the body. Also, try eating foods rich in B vitamins, such as whole grains, peanuts, bananas, and sunflower seeds, which help to counteract the effects of stress. On a side note, avoid alcohol. Alcohol can cause you to fall asleep quickly, but many people wake up in the middle of the night and have trouble getting back to sleep.

Cut out caffeine. Coffee, soft drinks, tea, and some medications are filled with caffeine, which can greatly interfere with a good night's sleep. If you must have coffee, reserve it for the early hours of the day, and then be caffeine free from noon until bedtime. Even one cup of coffee (150 milligrams of caffeine) can disturb the quality of sleep, increasing wakefulness and making it difficult to feel rested the next day.

Surprisingly, chocolate contains little caffeine. According to the International Food Information Council (IFIC) Foundation, an eight-ounce carton of chocolate milk contains about five milligrams of caffeine and an eight-ounce milk chocolate bar contains about forty milligrams of caffeine. An eight-ounce cup of regular coffee contains from eighty-eight to one hundred and sixty milligrams of caffeine, and an extrastrength Excedrin (one pill) has sixty-five milligrams of caffeine.

Take a warm bath before bedtime. Core body temperature has a twenty-four-hour rhythm that supplies the internal timing for sleep and wakefulness. Sleep characteristically occurs when the body temperature is declining, whereas wakefulness occurs when the temperature is rising. In findings published in April 2005 in the journal *Clinical and Sports Medicine,* researchers found that the skin temperature of hands and feet (particularly *warm feet*) seems to be the crucial variable for the association between internal body temperatures, sleepiness, and sleep. Because sleep usually follows the cooling phase of your body's temperature cycle, I recommend the practice of taking a shower or leisurely warm bath before bedtime. In addition, keep the temperature of your bedroom no higher than 68 degrees to induce this cooling phase associated with deep sleep. Another way to warm the body in preparation for deep sleep is to soak in a Jacuzzi before bedtime. The combination of heat and buoyancy causes blood vessels to dilate, lowering your blood pressure and speeding the flow of oxygen and nutrients to your muscles.

Beware of medications that can interrupt sleep. Any prescribed medication or drug that passes the blood-brain barrier has the potential to change the quality of sleep. For example, if you take a stimulant medication early in the day, it may influence your sleep hours later. Other medications that can affect sleep include over-the-counter and prescribed decongestants, theophylline, beta-blockers, corticosteroids, thyroxine, and bronchodilators, among others. Not only do anxiety and depression compromise quality sleep, but the medications prescribed for these mood disorders can result in sleep disorders. Antidepressants such as the selective serotonin reuptake inhibitors (SSRIs), like Paxil, Prozac, and Lexapro, are known to have an effect on sleep quality. If you are taking medication, talk to your doctor about any sleep concerns.

Spend time outdoors each day, especially during the morning hours, to keep your body's rhythms in harmony. Researchers have found that exposure to daylight and darkness regulates the body's natural secretion of melatonin. Melatonin belongs to a class of compounds called antioxidants, which are necessary to mop up injurious free radicals and prevent oxidation. We know that melatonin is secreted in smaller amounts in perimenopause and menopause, and some experts even hint that melatonin may be linked in some way to the initiation of menopause! The production of melatonin is acutely suppressed by light exposure. If you want to try the natural melatonin supplement, talk to your doctor to see if it might help your sleep.

3. Try Deep Abdominal Breathing to Calm Your Mind

Breathing is one of the few automatic activities of the body that we can consciously control. Mindful or deep abdominal breathing actually alters the body's psychological state, making a stressful moment diminish in intensity. Think about how your respiration quickens when you are fearful. Then consider how taking a deep, slow breath brings an immediate calming effect, reducing this stress. During deep abdominal breathing, you oxygenize the blood and trigger endorphins throughout the body while decreasing the release of stress hormones. Along with taking a warm bath or shower (page 111), studies show that relaxation techniques such as deep abdominal breathing help to induce distal vasodilation, a warming of the hands and feet, which is followed by sleep.

While lying in bed, you can use this sleep enhancer to slow your heart rate and calm your body. If you awaken during the night, immediately start your deep abdominal breathing to calm down and put your mind and body back into sleep mode.

To Do

- Lie on your back in a quiet room with no distractions.
- Place your hands on your abdomen and slowly inhale through your nostrils. If your hands are rising and your abdomen is expanding, then you are breathing correctly. If your hands do not rise and you see your chest rising, you are breathing incorrectly.
- Reposition yourself if you are breathing incorrectly and inhale slowly to a count of five, watching your hands rise over your abdomen. Pause for three seconds, and then exhale to a count of five, watching your hands descend with your abdomen.
- Start with ten repetitions of this exercise and increase to twenty-five reps twice daily. Use deep abdominal breathing any time you feel anxious, overwhelmed, or stressed. You can do this sitting up in your office chair, if needed, as long as you perform the breathing properly.

4. Lose Weight if Snoring Is a Problem

Snoring is a major sleep disrupter for men and women, especially after age forty. Two key risk factors for snoring in women are age (menopause) and being overweight or obese. You cannot change your age, but you can lose weight to decrease the chance of snoring and other problems associated with obesity.

5. Have a Consistent Bedtime Skin Ritual

- No matter how tired you are, always remove any makeup before bed.
- While lying in bed, avoid touching your face. This can exacerbate acne breakouts and irritate sensitive facial skin.
- Prop your head on two pillows at night to help ease under-eye circles. If you have neck problems, talk to your doctor and see if this is appropriate with your condition.
- Go easy on eye cream before bedtime, applying only a small dab underneath the eye. Make sure the cream does not spread into the eye to avoid irritation.
- Use a night cream that has moisturizing ingredients such as urea, hyaluronic acid, and sodium lactate.
- Consider using Renova, a vitamin A acid, if you have fine lines and blotchy skin. This prescription medication helps to fight wrinkles and smooth uneven skin tone. Unfortunately, many patients complain of irritation with products such as Renova, and any accrued skin benefits are reversible once treatment stops.

6. Have Regular Massages to Boost Sleep

As we discuss in Step 4, Relax, getting regular massages helps to increase relaxation, which can help to calm anxiety and improve sleep problems. In fact, some studies have shown that during a massage, the brain boosts the production of endorphins, chemicals that regulate the activity of a group of nerve cells in the brain that relax muscles, dull pain, and reduce panic and anxiety. Massage therapy may also trigger serotonin, a brain chemical that makes you feel calm and serene. It makes sense that when stress is alleviated, you can sleep peacefully.

7. Try Feng Shui for a Peaceful Sleep Environment

Feng shui is the ancient Chinese practice of placement of materials to achieve harmony with the environment. Using feng shui in the bedroom is said to balance Chi (energy) and improve the space as you prepare the mind and body for deep, healing sleep. Consider the following suggestions:

- Whether at work or at home, clutter has a strong negative impact on our mental and physical being. Clean out excess clutter in your bedroom, focusing on your closet, under the bed, and dresser, to aid relaxation at nighttime.
- Electromagnetic energy in the bedroom might result in poor health, according to feng shui practitioners. To keep your bedroom peaceful and a haven for rest, move the television, computer, radio, and answering machine to another room. If you want to keep electronics in the bedroom, place them at least six feet away from your bed.
- Have a healthy plant or two in the bedroom. Feng shui practitioners believe that plants absorb stress and have a positive impact on our healing process.
- As you prepare for bed, play soft music or a "sounds of nature" CD to create a tranquil, spa-like environment in the room.
- Feng shui practitioners believe that sharp edges or corners on walls, furniture, and rooflines are symbolic of poison arrows. Soften sharp corners in the bedroom by hanging a plant or wind chime from the ceiling.

Beyond Botox Recommendations for Rest

1. Find your sleep zone for sexy, ageless skin.
2. Plan a regular bedtime routine.
3. Try deep abdominal breathing to calm your mind.
4. Lose weight if snoring is a problem.
5. Have a consistent bedtime skin ritual.
6. Have regular massages to boost sleep.
7. Try feng shui for a peaceful sleep environment.

Chapter 7

Step #4: Relax

De-stress to Boost Skin Healing

When Karen's husband died suddenly several years ago, this forty-three-year old mother of two became the sole breadwinner for the family. At first, Karen found it challenging to be back in the business world, using her interior-design degree for the first time in two decades. Yet after months of raising kids alone, managing the household, and trying to make ends meet, she began to wear the stress of her frenetic lifestyle on her face.

When I met Karen in New York City in 2003, she desperately wanted advice on how to look relaxed — even if she didn't always feel relaxed. I sensed that this extremely thin and gaunt woman had been through a lot just from the signs of exhaustion on her face: the drab complexion, intense worry lines on her forehead, and the way her mouth seemed to draw downward as if in a perpetual frown. In talking with me, she said that the emotional stress of her husband's sudden death, along with the new position of parenting alone while working full-time, had resulted in daily tension, poor eating habits, and little sleep or time for herself.

"On most days, I'm so exhausted that I fall asleep on top of the bed without having dinner or even washing my face," Karen said.

Karen admitted that she felt trapped, with no time for herself, and she had recently started psychotherapy to gain some tools for making time to relax each day. I suggested that she also start the Beyond Botox seven-step program to learn some easy ways to pamper herself, care for her neglected skin, and reverse some of the visible lines and wrinkles that seemed to result from her harried lifestyle. Within four weeks of setting new priorities that included making time for herself and her skin, Karen wrote an e-mail to me and attached a snapshot — a photograph that showed a vibrant, attractive woman who appeared healthy and youthful again.

All Stressed Up

Stress. We live with it each day. For some of us, daily stress causes us to become irritable, short-tempered, or unable to concentrate on tasks. Others of us experience interrupted sleep, difficulty in falling asleep, or early-morning awakening. Then there are those of us who find that stress "gets under our skin" — we suffer with itchy or burning rashes, acne, rosacea, and other skin disorders. Although doctors have long maintained that stress affects immune function, it has only been in recent years that findings have indicated the effect of stress on the skin. These stresses can lead to premature aging of the skin in the form of fine lines, deeper wrinkles, and a dull complexion.

Whether they are juggling children, careers, or other daily commitments, women today are feeling the physical effects of stress and exhaustion. A revealing study conducted at the Behavioral Medicine Research Center at Duke University in Durham, North Carolina, found that working women with children at home create greater amounts of the stress hormone cortisol and experience higher levels of stress at home than those without children at home. Cortisol can sometimes help you perform well under pressure, but the resulting rise in testosterone increases the skin's oil production and can lead to acne and other breakouts. In your quest for healthy, ageless skin, chronic stress may well be your biggest obstacle, but it's one you can easily manage with some lifestyle changes.

In this chapter, I'll show you how daily stress results in physical exhaustion that depletes the skin of hydration, vitamin C, and oxygen; increases hormone levels and sebum (oil) production; and makes your skin look pale, tired, wrinkled, and old. Next, I will explain how the best deterrent to chronic stress is learning how to elicit the relaxation response at will to decrease the feeling of being all revved up. Along with meditation and some easy mind/body tools, I'll explain the various types of hands-on touch therapies such as Swedish massage that can help ease muscle tension and let you relax — instantly. Finally, I'll introduce our Beyond Botox program suggestions on how to de-stress daily by identifying your stress signals, learning to reconfigure your "to-do" list to allow time for yourself, and taking advantage of spa therapies, exercise, and yoga to keep your body in relaxation mode no matter what you face each day.

The Stages of Stress

Scientist Hans Selye was one of the first researchers to write about stress and its effect on the body. In 1926, Selye defined stress as "the nonspecific response of the body to any demand" and described the stages of stress, which he called the general adaptation syndrome (GAS), in his book *Stress Without Distress* (1974). Selye's three stages identify why stress can cause problems to the body. They are:

Stage 1: Alarm Reaction. Any physical, emotional, or mental upset will cause an instantaneous reaction by the body to combat the stressor. This physical response is well known as the "fight-or-flight" reaction. The fight-or-flight reaction sends a tremendous burst of adrenaline to all parts of the body. If the stress is acute, or short-term (in biological terms, short-term would be a few hours, perhaps even a couple of days), we quickly recover without any detrimental effect to the body. If the stress is chronic, or long-term, the body's resistance is affected, making us more susceptible to illness.

Stage 2: Resistance. At the resistance stage of chronic stress, the body tries to become balanced (a process called homeostasis). You may think you can handle anything because the stress symptoms noticed in the alarm stage have now calmed down — until you become completely exhausted. As the stress continues, you may suffer with fatigue, sleep problems, and overall malaise. If you get poor sleep, you may become quite irritable and have difficulty concentrating or being productive at home or work. This creates even more stress, and a vicious cycle has started.

Stage 3: Exhaustion. After combating stress for days to weeks, the body begins to shut down. Sometimes after days of unending stress, the body succumbs to illness, either a viral or bacterial infection. If you look back over a period of several years, you may find that the times you developed a cold or flu were immediately after stressful periods in your life.

It is during this exhaustion stage that your skin may pay the price. Chronic, or long-term, stress depletes the epidermis of water, oxygen, and vitamin C, as well as increases hormone levels, histamines, and sebum production. While completely unaware of the internal damage from chronic stress, you will notice how it manifests in skin symptoms such as bumps, excess oil, breakouts, acne, rosacea, pimples, and a host of other conditions.

Nagging daily stress also causes us to ignore good eating habits, as most people turn to fast foods, high-fat snacks, sugary desserts, and alcohol. When you combine poor diet, lack of sleep, and sedentary habits with chronic stress, perhaps it becomes clear how psychosocial stress directly influences skin aging and even skin disease.

The general adaptation syndrome makes it clear that stress affects the body, both initially and over a long period of time, but there are positive ways to respond to life's stressors so you do not experience immune dysfunction and the resulting skin problems and illness. Before you allow daily stress to cause unnecessary facial tension, frown lines, or skin eruptions, it is important to identify your personal stress response and consider changing your coping style.

Indirect Effects of Stress on Your Skin

Chronic stress can result in the following unhealthy habits that directly affect the skin:

Smoking
Sedentary lifestyle
Overuse of alcohol
Lack of sleep
Poor diet

The Pitfalls of Stress

Stress Shows on Your Skin

For years, scientists have focused on photoaging, cigarette smoking, and other lifestyle habits as determinant factors that contribute to premature skin aging. Yet some new findings underscore the prevalence of chronic (long-term) stress in activating premature skin aging and even skin cancer. In fact, in some patients, stress and sun may be a lethal combination.

In a study at Johns Hopkins Medical School, Dr. Francisco Tausk and his colleagues did a study seeking to establish a link between stress and skin cancer. While acute (short-term) stress actually boosts immune function, chronic (long-term) or daily stress appears to interrupt healthy skin function. Evidence from the past several decades suggests that emotional states such as depression, worrying, hostility, and psychosocial stress directly influence both body function and health.

As we learn more about the brain-skin interplay, we now believe that our mental state is closely related to skin function in humans. Along with skin cancer and premature skin aging, a large number of chronic skin diseases, including acne, rosacea, and atopic dermatitis, appear to be precipitated or exacerbated by psychological stress. This assumption was confirmed in findings published in the July 2003 issue of the journal *Archives of Dermatology,* when Dr. Susan Chon and colleagues at Stanford University concluded that emotional stress influenced the severity of acne. This connection had been long suspected (even now, don't you often see a pimple during particularly stressful times?), and these researchers found that patients with acne experienced a significant worsening during times of increasing stress.

Other dermatological studies have concluded the same: psychological stress has a significant and detrimental effect on treatment outcome in those individuals with problem skin.

Stress Shows in Your Health

Chronic or daily stress activates the sympathetic nervous system, stimulating the release of hormones such as cortisol (which we discussed earlier). But in addition to the negative effects excess cortisol can have on your skin, it can have far more serious effects on the rest of your body. A constant saturation of cortisol results in many physical changes in the body, including increased heart rate, respiration rate, and blood pressure. Under normal conditions these changes subside quickly, but chronic stressors, including anxiety, fear, anger, and grief, can keep the nervous system perpetually aroused.

Given the recent findings that show stress contributing to skin problems and diseases, it seems logical to presume that decreasing stress can decrease a person's susceptibility to and duration of illness. The most convincing evidence appears in two small but well-done studies by researchers at the UCLA School of Medicine, published in the *Archives of General Psychiatry*. The first study found that malignant melanoma patients trained in relaxation techniques showed significant increases in the number and activity of cancer-slaying natural killer cells. The second study, a recently published six-year follow-up, found higher mortality among the untrained group and those who did not use relaxation techniques.

Not only is stress uncomfortable, it is also linked to the following illnesses:

- Allergies, asthma, and hay fever
- Arthritis
- Back pain
- Cancer
- Chronic pain
- Heart disease
- High blood pressure
- Migraine headaches
- Temporomandibular joint (TMJ) syndrome
- Tension headaches
- Stroke
- Ulcers

Herbert Benson, MD, found in his studies that there is a counterbalancing mechanism to the fight-or-flight response. For instance, it is thought that stimulating an area of the hypothalamus in the brain can cause the stress response, and activating other areas of the brain results in the reduction of the stress response. Benson's work led to the discovery of what is called "the relaxation response," a physiological state of inner quiet and peacefulness and calming of negative thoughts and worries. (There are many techniques to elicit the relaxation response, which I explain later on.)

Relaxation is defined by decreased muscle tension and respiration, lower blood pressure and heart rate, and improved circulation. The relaxation response slows down the sympathetic nervous system, the "keyed-up" part of the autonomic nervous system that activates the secretion of epinephrine and norepinephrine. When the sympathetic nervous system slows down, you will experience the following:

- Decreased heart rate
- Decreased blood pressure
- Decreased sweat production
- Decreased oxygen consumption
- Decreased catacholamine production (dopamine and norepinephrine, brain chemicals associated with the stress response)
- Decreased cortisol (stress hormone) production

In this step, you will learn how to incorporate relaxation therapies into your daily regimen.

Take Your Skin Stress Quotient

Check each situation that you've experienced over the past few months that may have led to stress-related skin changes:

___ Work deadlines and pressures

___ Financial troubles

___ Job loss or insecurity

___ Chronic illness

___ Problems with marriage or other relationships

___ Caregiving to young children and/or aging parents

___ Personal turmoil and emotional upsets

___ Waiting in long lines of traffic

(continued)

— Juggling a career and raising children

— Specific worries about skin changes, including premature skin aging and/or skin cancer

If you checked even one or two of the above situations, you need to address the problem of stress in your life, and then start today to revamp your commitments and change the way you respond to life's interruptions.

The Relaxation Response

Most relaxation therapies are based on the premise that the mind and body are interconnected, and physical health and emotional well-being are closely linked. Not only can certain mind-body therapies increase the brain's morphine-like pain relievers, called endorphins and enkephalins, which are associated with a happy, positive feeling, these therapies may improve your quality of sleep, your ability to concentrate and be productive, and your personal relationships. One small study of several different relaxation modalities found a 42 percent improvement in self-reported sleep complaints after one year of practicing relaxation therapies. There are also fascinating reports that mind-body exercises used with touch therapies (bodywork and massage) are beneficial to psychological function, and the physiological benefits of these techniques extend for hours and even days.

Learn to Relax

Many women benefit from regular spa experiences, discussed in step 6, Pamper, as they relax with a Swedish massage or other touch therapies. I believe that eliciting the relaxation response in conjunction with massage is an effective way to reduce the emotional stress of daily living. Once you've learned the physiological process of relaxing (described below), no matter where you are — at work, at home, or traveling — you can elicit this decrease in sympathetic arousal with the various mind-body interventions, such as progressive muscle relaxation, meditation, guided imagery, and deep abdominal breathing.

To Do

1. Set aside a period of about fifteen to twenty minutes each day, and remove any outside distractions that can disrupt your concentration. Take the telephone off the hook or let your voice mail respond to incoming calls.

2. Recline comfortably on a bed, sofa, or floor so that your entire body is supported. Use a pillow or cushion under your head if this helps.

3. Remain calm and still. Focus your thoughts on the immediate moment and try to imagine that every muscle in your body is becoming loose, relaxed, and free of any tension.

4. Concentrate on making your breathing slow and even, breathing in a rhythmic fashion. As you exhale each breath, picture your muscles becoming even more relaxed, as if you are breathing the tension away.

5. At the end of the time period, focus on your relaxed state and notice whether any muscles that felt tight and tense initially now feel loose and relaxed.

If the relaxation response is practiced regularly, your body will learn to elicit it automatically, helping to relieve any anxiety that occurs. Many of our clients find that after several weeks of daily, consistent practice, they can maintain the relaxed state beyond the practice session itself.

Meditation

Meditation is an excellent mind-body therapy, as you focus your mind on one thought, phrase, or prayer for a certain period of time. Mindfulness meditation is a process of purposefully paying attention to what is happening in the present moment without being distracted by what has already happened or what might happen. When you do this, it leads to the relaxation response, which can help to decrease heart rate, blood pressure, respiratory rate, and muscle tension. Meditation also decreases hormones such as cortisol and adrenaline, which are released during the fight-or-flight, or stress, response, as discussed on page 118.

Meditation can guide you beyond the negative thoughts and agitations of the busy mind and allow you to become "unstuck" from fear and other disturbing emotions. Once you've learned how to meditate effectively, you can switch into this relaxation state at will — before stressors overwhelm you.

To Do

1. Sit in a comfortable chair in a quiet room. Make sure there are no distractions.

2. Close your eyes as you begin to meditate, and allow fifteen to twenty minutes for this exercise.

3. Focus your attention on the repetition of a word, sound, phrase, or prayer, doing this silently or whispering. An alternative is to focus on the sensation of each breath as it moves in and out of your body.

4. Each time your attention wanders (which will occur naturally), gently redirect it back. If you continue to practice this, you will learn how to do it correctly.

Progressive Muscle Relaxation

Progressive muscle relaxation is another stress reducer that can be done anytime. It involves contracting, then relaxing all the muscle groups in the body, beginning with your head and neck and progressing down to your shoulders, arms, hands, chest, back, stomach, pelvis, buttocks, legs, and feet.

To Do

1. Lie on your back in a quiet room with no distractions.

2. Starting with your forehead, focus on each set of muscles. Tense these muscles to the count of ten, then release to the count of ten. Feel the tension release as you let go of the muscle contraction.

3. Progress slowly downward and throughout your body, taking as long as you can to tense the muscles and release them. Get in touch with each body part and notice how it feels to be tense and then how it feels to be tension-free upon release of the muscle.

Visualization

Visualization, or guided imagery, has been used successfully for controlling emotional distress and anxiety. Ideally, you should use this therapy in a quiet environment without distractions. But it can also defuse a tense moment when you are in a confrontation at home or at work, while you're waiting on the telephone on hold, or while you're sitting in lines of rush-hour traffic.

To Do

1. Lie on your back or sit calmly in a comfortable chair. Initially, this should be learned in a quiet room with no distractions.

2. Visualize a peaceful, relaxing scene, perhaps a vacation spot you have enjoyed in the mountains or at the seashore. Blocking all other thoughts, focus on this peaceful retreat and try to recapture the moment as you imagine the sounds, smells, textures, and feelings you experienced.

3. Become aware of your breathing as you focus on the relaxing scene. Remember to breathe slowly from your abdomen, not your chest, inhaling to the count of five, holding for three seconds, and then exhaling to the count of five. Do not let outside stimuli interrupt your imagery time. Do this visualization exercise for ten to fifteen minutes whenever you need a break from your fast-paced routine.

Let Music Soothe the Soul

Studies show that listening to soothing music lowers blood pressure and boosts immune cell count while reducing levels of stress hormones. Reduced stress will result in less facial tension and smoother skin. Avoid melodies that make you tense or that cause uneasiness. Spend ten to twenty minutes a day listening to music, and try this in combination with another mind-body technique, such as guided imagery (visualization), deep abdominal breathing, or progressive muscle relaxation, or while you're walking outdoors or on a treadmill.

Bodywork and Touch Therapies

Bodywork (also called manual healing therapy) is an umbrella term that refers to a variety of body-manipulation therapies that aid in relaxation and rehabilitation. Massage therapy, the therapeutic manipulation of the body's soft tissues, is perhaps the most popular.

Although we cannot change life's stressors, studies indicate that we can use relaxation tools such as massage as a buffer during negative events. Massage therapy helps to ease pent-up tension, increase blood flow, and stimulate the flow of lymph (a bodily fluid that carries wastes and impurities away from tissues and that relies on muscle contractions to move efficiently through the body).

The fundamental medium of massage therapy is human touch. The various massage methods are described as a series of special techniques, but touch is not used solely in a mechanistic way. There is a great artistic component to the various manual techniques such as gliding, rubbing, kneading, tapping, manipulating, holding, friction pressure, and vibrating — using primarily the hands. Sometimes massage therapists use forearms, elbows, and even their feet as well. These techniques affect the musculoskeletal, circulatory-lymphatic, nervous, and other systems of the body.

There are more than a hundred different methods classified as massage therapy or bodywork, and approximately sixty of them are less than twenty years old. Swedish massage is the most popular, but other types are quickly growing in demand.

Special Caution for Women

Most doctors consider massage to be off-limits during the first trimester of pregnancy and to be used with extreme caution during the second and third trimesters. There is always the risk that pressure from massage may dislodge the baby or even induce labor. Also, though massage can help alleviate back pain and cramps during menstruation, the strokes and pressure have been found to increase menstrual flow. Talk to your doctor to see what's best for your situation.

Swedish massage. With Swedish massage, the practitioner uses a system of long strokes, kneading, and friction techniques to massage the more superficial layers of the muscles. This hands-on touch is combined with active and passive movements of the joints, and oil is usually used to stimulate metabolism and circulation. The therapist applies pressure and rubs the muscles in the same direction as the flow of blood returning to the heart. Swedish massage is said to help flush the tissues of lactic and uric acids and other metabolic wastes, as well as to improve circulation without increasing the load on the heart.

In a study published in the *International Journal of Neuroscience,* Tiffany Field and colleagues at the University of Miami Touch Research Institute found Swedish massage beneficial in reducing anxiety and enhancing alertness and math computation skills.

Neuromuscular massage. Neuromuscular massage combines the basic principles of Asian pressure therapies along with a specific

Self-Massage

You don't have to get a professional massage to benefit from touch therapy. If you have tension in your jaw, neck, or shoulders, you can massage these areas gently with your fingertips to ease tight muscles and decrease stiffness.

I. Use your favorite massage oil or cream. Take a few drops of the oil in your hand and gently touch the back of your neck, about two inches below the hairline, with your fingertips, rubbing the oil into the skin.

2. As you make contact with the skin, start using a circular motion with your fingertips, gently moving up and down the neck.

3. Work outward down the side of the neck to your shoulders, continuing the gentle circular motion.

4. Squeeze your shoulders one at a time using the opposite hand. Then, using long stroking motions, gently sweep the skin from the neck to the shoulder and down to the elbow.

5. If you suffer from carpal tunnel syndrome, gently massage the wrist and thumb areas to release tension there.

hands-on deep-tissue therapy to help reduce chronic muscle tension or myofascial (soft-tissue) pain.

Neuromuscular massage is applied specifically to individual muscles. It is used to increase blood flow, release trigger points (intense knots of muscle tension that refer pain to other parts of the body), and release pressure on nerves caused by soft tissues.

Deep-tissue massage. Deep-tissue massage is applied with greater pressure and at deeper layers of the muscle than Swedish massage and is used to release chronic patterns of muscular tension using slow strokes, direct pressure, or friction. Often the movements are directed across the grain of the muscles (cross-fiber) using the fingers, thumbs, or elbows.

Myofascial release. Myofascial release is a way of stretching tissue to make postural and alignment changes by releasing tension in the fascia. The fascia is fibrous connective tissue that gives strength and support to the body. But when the fascia becomes constricted due to aging, illness, or trauma, it can become tight and pull muscles or bones out of alignment. This form of bodywork is particularly helpful in reducing muscle tension and easing chronic stress.

The Trager method. Unlike massage, Trager avoids pressure, using gentle, rhythmic rocking and shaking to release tension and loosen joints. During the session, the practitioner moves the client's trunk and limbs in a gentle, rhythmic way so that the person experiences new sensations of freedom of movement. The practitioner's

Is Your Massage Therapist Licensed?

The licensing of massage therapists varies from state to state. The American Massage Therapy Association is the largest national professional organization of bodyworkers. Membership requires training at an accredited school and hundreds of hours of supervised practice. The National Certification Board for Therapeutic Massage and Bodywork (NCBTMB) requires practitioners to adhere to a set of standards that outlines acceptable behaviors. Make sure you feel comfortable with the practitioner you choose.

Nadia's Healing Massage

Extensive studies have shown that massage in particular reduces anxiety and lowers the body's production of stress hormones. That healing response gives a significant benefit to someone like forty-nine-year-old Nadia, the manager of a chain of office supply stores based in Brooklyn, New York, who could not get relief from chronic stress associated with her job.

When I went to the appointment at a nearby massage therapy center, I was impressed at how professional everyone was. The receptionist asked me to fill out a medical-history form, and then one of the therapists took me into a small room that was painted a very soothing blue. There was classical music playing in the background, and aromatherapy candles were burning near the window-sill. The therapist showed me to a dressing area, where I exchanged my street clothes for a long white sheet, which I discreetly tucked around my body.

I sat on the long table, and the therapist began to rub sweet-smelling sesame oil on my skin, then she softly kneaded my tightened muscles. Using a gentle rocking motion, the therapist began to release tension out of my upper body, and then had me lie down facing the table. Her hands worked up and down the painful trigger points on my back, shoulders, and thighs. Sometimes I felt like her fingers were pointing right into my skin, but she said that was where my muscles were extremely tense. She focused mostly on my upper body — my neck, shoulders, and upper back — where my pain was the worst.

After the massage, I was almost afraid to move. I was relaxed, and the muscle tension was almost nonexistent. Finally, as I was getting dressed, I realized that the range of motion in my arms was greater and the tightness in my upper body was greatly reduced. I continued receiving thirty-minute massages once a week for several months and had greatly reduced muscle tension and stiffness, less fatigue, and was able to sleep for seven hours a night. I became more effective on the job and at home because of taking time for a weekly massage.

goal is to help the client really feel what relaxation should be like. Trager therapists believe that the resulting deeply relaxed feelings can resonate through the nervous system, ultimately benefiting tissues and organs deep within the body.

Putting the Program into Action

Relax for Sexy, Ageless Skin

Your particular patterns of muscle tension are learned responses, not part of your genetic makeup. In other words, each time life's stressors hit, we all respond differently, whether by pursing our lips, clenching our jaw, or furrowing our brow — and all of these facial expressions can result in permanent wrinkles over time. The real problem is that chronic stress can trigger premature skin aging. You can reverse this pattern by relearning how to respond to your stressors in a healthy manner.

1. Identify Your Skin Stress Symptoms

How does your skin respond to stress? Some women break out in hives: others have exacerbations of acne or rosacea. Review the following list of skin stress signs and symptoms, as well as other physical and emotional symptoms of stress, and check those that apply to you:

Skin Stress Symptoms

Acne	Oily skin
Dry, itchy skin	Pimples flare
Eczema	Rashes
Fever blister on lips	Rosacea
Hives	Under-eye circles from lack of sleep

Other Physical and Emotional Symptoms:

Anger	Inability to concentrate
Anxiety	Insomnia
Apathy	Irregular menstrual periods
Back pain	Loss of sexual desire
Chest pain or tightness	Mood swings
Colitis	Neck pain
Depression	No energy
Headaches	Rapid pulse
Heart palpitations	Short temper
Irritable bowel syndrome (IBS)	Short-term memory loss
Impotence	Weight gain or loss
Inability to relax	

Now, as you become aware of your responses to stress during daily activities, use the following technique to react positively:

1. *Stop* when stressors begin to make you feel anxious and overwhelmed.

2. *Breathe* from your abdomen, inhaling to the count of five, holding to the count of three, and exhaling to the count of five.

3. *Relax* your muscles throughout your body as you try to change your response.

4. *Mindfully* focus on a relaxing scene as you try to change your mind's perception and switch into the relaxation response.

2. Cross One Item Off Your "To Do" List

As you seek to control your stress response, it's important to look at your "to do" list to avoid becoming overly committed. Especially if you are balancing career, children, and other commitments, you should not feel guilty about prioritizing what is humanly possible.

Write down the tasks that face you each day. As you schedule your day, budget ample time to get your work completed by calculating how long a project will take you, then adding an extra fifteen to thirty minutes to allow yourself to go at a more moderate speed instead of always dashing in high gear. This will cut you some leeway, especially on those busy days when life's stressors hold you back from optimum performance.

If you find that you have more tasks scheduled than time available, rewrite your list and prioritize the projects you must do, putting the less-important projects or activities at the bottom of the list. These can always wait until another day, or you can delegate them to others. Sharing the load is crucial as you learn to balance your day, doing what your body will let you do without excessive stress or fatigue.

Some women prefer to make their "to do" lists each morning. Others find that writing the "to do" list the night before relieves their minds and enables them to sleep better.

Take time weekly to evaluate your commitments and focus on those that are most important, saying no to the remaining tasks. Saying no, when appropriate, can bring your stress to a manageable level and give you some control over your life. Also, when you successfully follow through with your commitments, you can reduce unnecessary pressure.

Other de-stressing tips include:

- On the job, organize your work before you do anything else. Write down a list of priorities for the day and keep these next to your workstation. Check off each task as you complete it so you feel a sense of accomplishment.
- Delegate responsibilities at home and at work.
- Realize that it's okay to be "good enough." When the pressure cooker of life begins to explode, remember that you are one person. We can do the best possible, or be "good enough," but we also have to realize our humanness and allow for this.
- Stop multitasking. This is a trend among many today, and it will only add to your list of stressors. Do one thing at a time and mindfully focus on what you're doing. You will get more accomplished because you do it right the first time.
- Keep track of the fruits and vegetables you eat each day and aim to add a few more (Step 1, Nourish). Doing something you know is good for your body can give you added confidence during stressful times.
- Add time for movement each day, but do not be obsessive (Step 2, Move). Studies are now suggesting that exercise is even better than some pills for fighting anxiety and depression.
- Schedule time to get ample sleep, as discussed in Step 3, Rest. Sleep deprivation is a stressor in itself, as deep sleep is neces-

sary for restoring energy so that you can handle life's interruptions effectively.

3. Plan Daily Time-Outs to Relax

To begin your relaxation program, set aside a period of about fifteen minutes that you can devote solely to relaxation practice. Choose a time when you have few obligations or commitments, so you won't feel rushed. Remove outside distractions that can disrupt your concentration: turn off the radio, the television, even the ringer on the telephone. Try each of the relaxation therapies in this step, and find the ones that work best for you. Alternatively, use each of them at various times of the day or week.

4. Schedule a Massage

Dana is a stay-at-home mom who manages the household and also helps out with her husband's business. Problem is, this thirty-four-year-old woman never takes time for herself. As her children have become older and more active, having no time for relaxation directly influences her patience and energy level.

The best way women can care for others is to first care for themselves. On her birthday last year, Dana's mother gave her a multiple-visit gift certificate to a day spa on Long Island, New York. Since incorporating a biweekly massage into her hectic schedule, Dana has more energy, patience, and strength, and her moods are much improved. No longer is she the harried mom who is continuously on the go. She seems to have a more positive attitude and clearer focus on what matters most in life. Dana says that taking that one hour to relax and care for herself has helped her become more organized and improved her outlook on life.

You don't have to wait for someone else to offer you a gift certificate to start taking better care of yourself. Find out what helps you disconnect from daily stress and allow yourself to let go, even just for an hour.

5. Give Yourself a Hand Massage

Keep a gentle moisturizing hand lotion on your desk. After rubbing the lotion into your hands, use one of your thumbs to press the area between the other thumb and forefinger. Breathe deeply for two minutes during this massage. Now reverse hands and do the same again.

6. Consider Yoga

Yoga uses stress-reduction techniques with gentle stretching and other positions to send fresh blood to muscles and internal organs, supplying them with nutrients and oxygen. This ancient Eastern discipline increases relaxation, reduces blood pressure, and relieves mental tension. In a study published in the journal *Work*, researchers found that regularly practicing yoga on the job helps employees improve work performance by relieving tension and job stress. It is thought that yoga may positively affect levels of body chemicals such as cortisol and other stress hormones, melatonin, and monoamines. Substantial research exists that supports the use of yoga for increasing intuition, perception, and attention.

7. Hit the Gym

If you are a chronic worrier, you may want to try exercising more often — and regularly. In findings presented in June 2002 at the American Psychological Society's annual meeting, researchers concluded that chronic worriers who exercised appeared to be less likely to suffer depressive symptoms than nonexercisers. Although the study was performed on students during final-exam week, researchers affirmed that the findings should apply to all worriers — and exercise is the treatment.

A chronic worrier is someone who worries about every situation in life: work, family, recreation activities, and more. You can block the effect worry has on your health — and skin — by doing something positive, like working out at the gym. Not only will exercise ease your emotional anxiety, it will help boost blood flow throughout your body, resulting in optimal health and healing for your immune system and your skin.

8. Laugh More

During stressful times, rent some funny videos and watch these instead of the nightly news. You'll sleep better after a good laugh, and it may help boost human growth hormone and a host of other healing chemicals in the body. An interesting Canadian study found that even looking forward to laughter improves immune function and decreases the effect of stress on the body. Humor therapy, laughter therapy, and comedy clubs all appear to have unique implications in reducing stress, reducing blood pressure, and improving immunity.

*   *   *

As you move to Step 5, Super-Saturate, remember to incorporate relaxation therapies throughout each day to successfully combat the chronic stress that can trigger premature skin aging and skin cancer, as well as exacerbate problems like rosacea, acne, and itchy rashes or hives. When these techniques are used in tandem with the daily strategies given in Steps 1 through 3, you will begin to enjoy the immediate physiological and psychological benefits that result in sexy, ageless skin.

Beyond Botox Recommendations for Relax

1. Identify your stress signals.
2. Check your "to do" list.
3. Plan daily time-outs.
4. Schedule a massage.
5. Give yourself a massage.
6. Consider yoga.
7. Hit the gym.
8. Laugh more.

Chapter 8

Step #5: Super-Saturate

Moisturize Properly to Quench Your Skin's Thirst

After using the same body moisturizer for more than two decades, Wendy, age fifty-four, realized that it was doing nothing to hydrate her skin. She was midflight on the way to her daughter's college graduation in Denver, Colorado, when she glanced down at her arms and noticed that the skin was dry and flaky and looked as if she had not moisturized it in weeks. She quickly coated her hands and arms in lotion from the small tube she kept in her purse, but in less than an hour the skin on her arms was dry and scaly again.

The next week, Wendy talked with her dermatologist, who said that the reduction in estrogen at menopause was the primary cause of her dramatic skin changes. The doctor commented on how dry and scaly Wendy's skin appeared and suggested that she use a more concentrated multipurpose antioxidant barrier-repair cream. Within a few weeks, Wendy saw a definite improvement in her skin texture and continues to moisturize several times daily to keep her skin supple and smooth.

*　　*　　*

So much myth and misinformation surround the understanding and treatment of skin changes with aging, and much of this is simply because of lack of knowledge. We find that most women are completely unaware of their particular skin needs, not to mention what the ingredients in the frequently advertised moisturizers they rub on their face and body can and cannot do. Many women don't know, for

example, that commonly used ingredients such as retinol (a derivative of vitamin A) can aggravate and even worsen skin conditions —
even when the advertisement claims "safe for sensitive skin." The
wrong moisturizer on your type of skin can do more harm than
good.

Years ago, when trying to better understand the principles of
skin hydration, I did an experiment in the laboratory that really
showed me how important it is to treat the skin, not just the symp-
tom. I took a small amount of tissue from a patient's callus and
divided it into two parts. One part was immersed in a sealed jar of
oil, and the other part in a sealed jar of water. After seventy-two
hours, I opened the jars and noted in my lab journal that the callus
tissue in oil remained hard and rigid, while the tissue in water
appeared soft and pliable. After keeping the water-immersed tissue
in the open air for eight hours, I noted that it had lost its pliability
and moisture and returned to its initial rigid state.

This experiment reinforced the notion that the simple application of water or oil is *not* the cure for dry skin. The real scientific
need is to find the specific ingredients for your skin type that will
mimic the natural moisturizing capabilities of healthy, young skin.

Knowing what ingredients to look for in skin care products can
help you achieve spectacular therapeutic effects. An example of this
is simple petrolatum, which is used in both pharmaceutical and cosmetic products. Petrolatum is a safe, nonirritant, noncomedogenic
emollient skin conditioner, especially beneficial for use on drier skin
types. Other helpful ingredients are ceramides, cholesterol, and
sodium PCA.

I talked a bit in chapter 3 about ingredients you should look
for in topical skin treatments like creams, moisturizers, and sunscreens. In this chapter, I go one step further and teach you how
to properly use moisturizing creams and lotions for maximum
benefit — no matter what your skin type. I'll briefly introduce you to
the specific skin types and teach you why you must first identify
your skin type before deciding which ingredients are most healing
(and which ones might be irritating). I'll also teach you how to select
the perfect moisturizer and then how to get the most out of moisturizing your skin (an easy technique I call "soak and super-saturate").
Finding the right sunscreen is a problem for most women, and I'll
talk about the importance of sunscreen, when to apply it and how

often, and how to select the proper sun-protection factor (SPF) for your skin type. Finally, as you start the Beyond Botox program, I'll teach you how to develop your own skin care regimen that includes cleansing, toning, exfoliating, and hydrating and moisturizing, and results in sexy, ageless skin.

Why *Super*-Saturate?

So far in the Beyond Botox seven-step program, I have discussed how certain nutrients, moderate exercise, healing sleep, and de-stressing all work together to help boost immune function and fight the injurious free radicals that are implicated as a cause of skin aging and disease. In this chapter, I will give you the most essential secret to sexy, ageless skin, and that is to *moisturize, moisturize, moisturize!*

In more clinical terms, I call this step "super-saturate" because water is an essential constituent of healthy skin. I want you to understand how excessive water loss (or gain) upsets the skin's physiology and function, and how you can compensate for this on a daily basis through the judicious use of moisturizers and other lubricants.

In normal, healthy skin, hydration proceeds from the inside out. But when skin lacks adequate hydration, it becomes brittle and flaky, looks extremely wrinkled, and undergoes other changes indicating that it is "thirsty." Without adequate moisture, skin looks old and dry, not vibrant and not sexy!

When excessive water in the dermal tissue is lost from the skin by evaporation, there must be a plan for replenishment. Our Beyond Botox plan involves an understanding of moisturizers and how they function, knowledge of your specific skin type and its needs, a regular regimen of cleansing the skin twice daily, and super-saturating with the finest moisturizers that meet your skin's particular needs.

Watch Out: Commonly Used Ingredients Can Irritate Skin

The following chemicals used in some cosmeceuticals may result in skin irritation. Always read the package label and check the ingredients before you rub anything on your skin.

- tretinoin (vitamin A acid)
- retinol (vitamin A alcohol)
- propylene glycol
- capsaicin
- camphor
- cinnaminic acid
- oil of bergamot
- ylang-ylang oil
- benzoin
- Peru balsam
- collodion

How Should I Choose a Moisturizer?

Before you choose a moisturizer, it's important to carefully assess your skin type. For instance, our client Kit (age thirty-two) was using the wrong moisturizer for years, and it was wreaking havoc with her skin. Kit has ultradry skin and pimples. Before understanding the proper type of moisturizer for her skin type, Kit said she used thick moisturizers for dry skin, which collected on dead skin cells, clogged her pores, and resulted in pimple breakouts. She was relieved to learn that simply selecting the proper moisturizer for her dry skin would alleviate her breakouts.

Once you learn all you can about your personal skin care needs, and with a greater understanding of specific ingredients in popular moisturizers, you can find the perfect one that treats your skin without causing flare-ups of pimples, acne, or rosacea. Here are some recent e-mails from clients who express concern in selecting the proper moisturizer.

Suzanne, a thirty-seven-year-old mother and senior editor of a well-known health magazine based in California, wrote to us for some answers to her moisturizing concerns.

> I've had oily skin and occasional acne as long as I can remember. Over the past year, my skin has become drier to the point that it is scaly and flakes off. The acne breakouts are less frequent, but if I use the wrong moisturizer, they come back with a vengeance. I religiously read labels so I know what ingredients I'm putting on my skin. Still, that does not guarantee a great product. Can you help me pick a specialized product that meets the needs of my particular skin?

Fifty-seven-year-old Paula from Chicago sent us the following e-mail, requesting a helpful chart so she could judiciously choose the best moisturizer.

> As a recent transplant from sunny south Florida to the suburbs of Chicago, I'm at a loss for how to best treat my skin. In south Florida, my normal/combination skin gave me no problems as long as I kept it lightly moisturized and used sunscreen daily. However, with the drier skin from menopause, combined with constant chafing from Chicago's very cold winters and blistering winds, my face stays inflamed, blotchy, and chapped no matter how I treat it.
>
> What can I use to calm my skin? What do I use when the summer months come and I don't need a heavy moisturizer?

Thirty-six-year-old Erin from Bangor, Maine, attached a picture with her e-mail. This attractive, outdoorsy woman looked as if she had rosacea with her bright red cheeks.

> As a lifelong resident of Bangor, Maine, I try to get out-of-doors as much as I can. While I teach year-round at the University of Maine, during the summer months, I enjoy boating with my friends and family. During the winter, I'm on the slopes at nearby resorts. The problem is my skin is always ruddy, rough, and dry. When I use moisturizers on my cheeks, it stings and seems to worsen the redness. If I don't

use a moisturizer, my skin peels and looks damaged. I know I need a specific program to get my skin back in shape. Can you advise me of the best treatments?

We explained to Suzanne, Paula, and Erin how to treat their specific skin conditions, using the information in this book. We also encouraged them to "type" their skin, meaning to find the exact type of skin they had. Once they did this, we guided them in selecting the perfect combination of ingredients for that skin type (see page 143).

Beyond Botox Moisturizing Guide

Because moisturizing preparations often contain multifunctional ingredients, it is difficult to attribute exact benefits to a specific component of a blended product. Using the table below, you can assess the different types of moisturizers and review the comments on their actions and uses for the skin.

Action	How it works	What it is used for	Examples
Emollient	Softens and smoothes skin	Decreases dry, rough skin	Petrolatum, squalane, lanolin, octyl dodecanol, isopropyl palmitate, isopropyl myristate, hexyl laureate, vegetable oils, glyceryl esters, and silicon oils
Occlusive	Slows water loss and conserves and increases the skin's moisture	Prevents itching, atopic dermatitis, and contact dermatitis	Petrolatum, zinc oxide, lanolin, mineral oil
Humectant	Attracts water to the stratum corneum	Prevents dry skin	Glycerin, lactic acid, sodium lactate, propylene glycol, Bio-Maple, urea, alpha hydroxy acid (AHA)

(continued)

Action	How it works	What it is used for	Examples
Film Former	Prevents trans-epidermal water loss (TEWL)	All skin types	Water-soluble silicone polymer, dimethicone, cyclomethicone, polyvinylpyrrolidone (PVP)
Lubricant	Prevents skin drying and irritation	Normal to dry skin types	Petrolatum, mineral oil, vegetable oils

Find Your Skin Type

Your skin type is a combination of three factors:

1. Water content, which is responsible for skin's suppleness
2. Lipid content, which is responsible for nutrition and softness
3. Level of sensitivity, which is responsible for the skin's resistance and tolerance

Using the following list, find your skin type. Once you've determined your skin type, read further to understand how to keep it balanced.

Normal Skin

___ Balanced sebaceous secretions
___ Slight shine on T zone
___ Possibility of a few comedones
___ Even texture, smooth to the touch
___ Pores visible but not dilated

Dry Skin

___ Insufficient sebaceous secretions
___ Thin skin

___ Cheeks drier than T zone
___ An uncomfortable pulling sensation
___ Fine lines
___ Matte complexion
___ Sensitive to environmental factors

Oily Skin

___ Excessive sebaceous secretions
___ Thicker texture
___ Shiny complexion
___ Oily to touch
___ Acneic tendency comedones

Normal Skin

Normal skin has barely visible pores, an even, smooth tone, soft texture, and no visible blemishes or flaky patches. The skin surface is supple and springy, and it is neither greasy nor dry. Because of the balanced amount of water and lipids and good blood circulation, normal skin appears to have few imperfections.

Skin goals for normal skin: Maintain, moisturize, protect. Normal skin still needs special attention to ensure that it remains balanced. It is important to use products that do not upset this balance, meaning they do not irritate, dehydrate, or increase photosensitivity. Look for ingredients such as petrolatum, mineral oil, silicone polymer, dimethicone, cyclomethicone, and polyvinylpyrrolidone (PVP).

Dry Skin

Dry skin has almost invisible pores and can be dull, rough, scaly, and itchy or thin and delicate. Dry skin can occur anywhere on the body, and of the three layers of skin, the epidermis is the main concern with dry skin.

Most people think that dry skin is caused by a lack of natural oils, but this is not the case. Dry, scaly skin is usually caused by an abnormal shedding of cells from the outer layer of the skin. Lubrication by the body's natural oils (sebum) or topical products helps to prevent water loss, but the skin must be hydrated first in order for these substances to be effective.

Dry skin can occur with aging, frequent bathing, hot showers or baths, high temperatures, and low humidity. Soaps, even those that are pure and mild, can worsen dry skin because excessive washing or scrubbing can also increase dryness.

The tendency to have dry skin is usually genetic. Dry skin also occurs with aging and environmental variations. Many women have dry skin during the hot summer months, but it is probably more common during the cold winter months, when humidity is low and heaters force dry air into enclosed rooms.

Skin goals for dry skin: Treat, nourish, and protect. It's important to keep dry skin well hydrated all the time by avoiding dry heat, hot showers and baths, rough clothing, and irritating cleansing products. Because bath soaps can strip the natural lipids from the skin, leaving it flaky, scaly, and cracked, use a moisturizing soap-lotion in a liquid form. In addition, super-saturate with a moisturizer immediately after bathing, while the skin is still damp. In some cases, oatmeal baths are helpful when skin is extremely dry.

During the winter months, cold air, dry wind, and low humidity combine to increase evaporation and reduce sweating, which results in dry, chapped skin that flakes, cracks, and even bleeds. To add moisture to the air, use a humidifier in your home or at least in your bedroom while you are sleeping. Be sure to clean the humidifier basin regularly to keep mold and mildew from breeding.

Check your diet to see if you are getting plenty of essential fatty acids, as discussed in Nourish. Avoid the sun and stay out of smoke-filled rooms. Smoking causes vasoconstriction (narrowing of the blood vessels) and decreases oxygen and other nutrients supplied by the capillaries in the skin.

To moisturize dry skin, look for products that have ingredients such as glycerin, lactic acid, sodium lactate, urea, alpha hydroxy acids, petrolatum, squalane, lanolin, and vegetable oils.

Normal Combination Skin

Almost three-fourths of the population has normal combination skin. This means they are usually normal to dry around their temples and on their cheeks, with an oily T zone. The pores of normal combination skin are large, and the skin tends to have blackheads. This skin type is often either overly dry or excessively oily, and the cheeks can appear rough. Depending on the time of year, the oiliness and dryness can change too. The skin is usually drier when the weather is cold, and even oily skin can become rough and irritated in winter.

Goals for normal combination skin: Balance, control oil, protect. Since combination skin means there are two competing skin types, it may be necessary to use more than one skin care product to achieve your goals. Milky-textured cleansers can rid the skin of excess oil without dehydrating the cheek area. These types of cleansers will give the skin a squeaky-clean feel while leaving it supple and soft. Using a combination skin toner under a lightweight moisturizer will help control oil and shine, bind moisture to the skin where it is needed, and also protect the skin from sun damage.

While normal combination skin is easy to care for, be sure to use ingredients such as petrolatum, mineral oil, vegetable oils, silicone polymer, dimethicone, cyclomethicone, and polyvinylpyrrolidone (PVP).

Oily Skin

Oily skin has dilated pores, a shiny complexion, blackheads, and pimples. Because hormones affect oil production, any factor that affects hormone levels (such as age, stress, or birth control pills) can also affect the skin.

Acne, a skin condition characterized by whiteheads, blackheads, and inflamed red pimples, or "zits," is often the result of oily skin. Acne occurs when pores on the surface of the skin become clogged. This happens when oil glands overproduce oil, resulting in pores blocked with dirt, bacteria, and debris.

Skin goals for oily skin: Control oil, hydrate, protect. Oily skin usually causes acne problems for teenagers, but this skin type is actually a plus for aging skin. However, it is important to use oil-free moisturizers because even oily skin requires moisture.

To keep oily skin healthy and youthful, use ingredients such as water-soluble silicone polymer, dimethicone, cyclomethicone, and polyvinylpyrrolidone (PVP).

What's in a Product Label?

- *Natural* simply means that the ingredients are not synthetic. Natural ingredients may include both animal and plant compounds.
- *Organic* means at least 95 percent of the ingredients are organically grown.
- *Not tested on animals* means the ingredient was not tested on animals (the same might not be true of the finished product).
- *Hypoallergenic* means a reduced potential of the product's triggering an allergic reaction, but there still may be some reaction.
- *Fragrance-free* means the product has no added fragrances. It could have natural fragrances from various ingredients.

How Much Sunscreen Do I Need?

No discussion of slathering your skin would be complete without a discussion of sunscreen and sun protection. No matter where you live, it is vital to understand the dangers of tanning, especially with the latest warnings (published in the August 2005 issue of the *Journal of the American Medical Association*) showing that the incidence of two types of skin cancer has nearly tripled among women under age forty. I mentioned the link between a fatty diet and skin cancer in Step 1, Nourish. But these findings confirm what I have been saying, that 80 percent of skin aging is a direct result of overexposure to the sun. The use of facial treatments such as baby oil, iodine, and sun reflectors by baby boomers during their teenage years now shows on their skin.

It's important for all women to know how to protect themselves from photoaging and skin cancer by selecting the sunscreen that best fits their skin type and lifestyle. Sunscreens constitute the mainstay of sunburn prevention. These topical agents protect the skin by absorbing, scattering, or reflecting ultraviolet radiation and visible light.

UVB rays cause the most immediate damage to the skin, resulting in sunburn and even cancer. The UVB rays penetrate the first layer of skin (epidermis) and trigger the cells that produce melanin, which then results in a dark complexion (or blistering sunburn). A product's sun protection factor (SPF) is defined as the ratio of the least amount of UVB energy required to produce a minimum erythema (redness) reaction after sunscreen application, as compared to the amount of energy required to produce the same reaction without a sunscreen. For instance, if it takes you ten minutes to develop redness after sun exposure and you apply a sunscreen with an SPF of 15, theoretically you should be protected approximately fifteen times your ten-minute exposure, or about a hundred fifty minutes, before you might develop the same level of skin redness. A sunscreen's effectiveness will depend on various factors, such as skin thickness and type (fair, olive, or black complexion), the time of day, and even your state of health. Medications can increase photosensitivity. Specific classes of photosensitizing drugs include antibiotics, birth control pills, diabetic medication, diuretics, tranquilizers, and antidepressants. In addition, topical therapies such as Retin-A and Renova can increase sensitivity to the sun's rays. Talk to your doctor about ways to protect your more sensitive skin if you use these.

As a chemist, I'm extremely concerned about cosmetics with SPF, especially foundation creams and lotions. There is a tendency among users to overestimate the effectiveness of the sun protection in these products, and they think they can skip a separate application of sunscreen just because their foundation contains some sun protection. Some women would rather not apply sunscreen because it is "greasy" or because it might mess up their makeup. The solution is to use cosmetically elegant sunscreen preparations, which may be applied both under and over makeup several times daily. These products are available and should be used regularly to prevent skin damage.

How to Use Sunscreen Effectively

1. Apply sunscreen daily at least twenty minutes before sun exposure.

2. Reapply every two hours, especially after swimming or excessive perspiration.

3. Apply sunscreen generously over all your exposed skin and be uniform with the application.

Beyond Botox Sunscreen Chart

Check the following chart to determine the SPF that is best for your skin, and *never* go outside without applying sunscreen.

Skin Type	Characteristics	SPF Recommendation
Type I	Always burns, never tans (i.e., extremely sensitive)	SPF of 45 or more
Type II	Always burns, sometimes tans (i.e., very sensitive)	SPF of 30 or more
Type III	Sometimes tans, sometimes burns (i.e., sensitive)	SPF of 30 or more
Type IV	Always tans, sometimes burns (i.e., minimally sensitive)	SPF of 15 or more
Type V	Always tans, never burns (i.e., not sensitive)	SPF of 15 or more
Type VI	Black skin (i.e., not sensitive)	SPF of 15 or more

Putting the Program into Action

Super-Saturate for Sexy, Ageless Skin

As you start to Super-Saturate for sexy, ageless skin, it is important to read the various tips in each category and then review the corresponding charts. This will enable you to fully understand the purpose of the action, whether cleansing, toning, exfoliating, or hydrating and moisturizing, among others.

1. Follow a Consistent Regimen for Sexy, Ageless Skin

Cleanse and Tone. It is important to cleanse your skin every night to remove makeup, impurities, dead skin cells, and excess oil. But a morning cleansing is also beneficial, as it removes any toxins the skin eliminates during the night and refreshes the skin, preparing it for makeup application.

For the removal of eye makeup, especially waterproof mascara, there are particular products specifically formulated for the eye area. However, some gentle facial cleansers can effectively remove all makeup, eye and facial, as well as cleanse the skin. When choosing a general, or "all-in-one," cleanser, be sure that it is fragrance- and color-free to avoid irritating the eye area. If you do not need to remove eye makeup, select a skin-specific cleanser. For instance, use an oil-free cleanser for oily skin, and a milky or creamy cleanser for drier skin.

The main use of a toner is to return the skin's pH to normal. It is also useful to complete the cleansing process, as it will remove any last traces of makeup and cleanser residue. Some toners have very beneficial ingredients that help certain skin conditions. As an example, ethanol will help with excess oil, and lactic acid or other alpha hydroxy acid (AHA) will help exfoliate and smooth the skin's texture.

Repair. There are specific types of products that treat or repair the skin, including serums, concentrate boosters, revitalizers, reparative products, and remedies. These products are usually independent of skin type and effectively treat skin conditions such as rosacea or hypersensitive skin, acne, hormone-deprived skin, dull complexions, dehydrated skin, pigmentary stains, and scarring.

Before selecting a product to treat a skin condition, it is a good idea to have professional advice to assess and diagnose the problem. This assessment should include a brief history of your health problems, medications you take, and any previous treatments. An experienced skin care professional should be able to assist you in selecting the appropriate therapy. One application of a treatment usually won't bring any significant results, but regular, consistent use can help. Since specific therapies usually have higher concentrations of ingredients, the products are often applied after cleansing.

Moisturize. When you hydrate your skin, you simply add water to it. To moisturize, you can add water, oil, or both.

The skin needs to be moisturized morning and evening, and it is important that the appropriate types of moisturizers are used to avoid aggravating any skin conditions. Refer to the discussion on page 142 to find the moisturizing ingredients that are right for your particular skin type.

Always apply moisturizers after cleansing and after any reparative treatment has been used unless otherwise indicated. Use my technique of "soak and super-saturate" for best results.

Protect from the sun. Protecting the skin daily with sunscreen helps guard it from the sun and other environmental factors. If your moisturizer has SPF, you do not need to add a sunscreen. If your day moisturizer does not have SPF, then use a sunscreen/sunblock on top of it. More and more cosmetic companies are formulating makeup such as foundation and powder that has SPF and may offer some sun protection. Powder makeup can also contain minerals that are physical sunscreens and offer some protection as well.

No matter what product you use, the skin must be protected from the sun to avoid photoaging, including age spots, premature aging, and sunburns, and the best way to accomplish this is to apply a sunscreen product that has been properly tested to offer both UVA and UVB protection.

Beyond Botox Four-Step Process for Sexy, Ageless Skin

1. Cleanse and Tone
2. Repair
3. Moisturize
4. Protect from the Sun

See Appendix II for more detailed information.

> ## Ultradry Skin Aids
>
> If your skin is ultradry during winter months, consider buying a humidifier for your home or bedroom to add extra moisture to the air. Also, bathe only every other day to retain the skin's natural oils. Avoid steamy baths or showers, which strip the skin's oily layer. Avoid using overefficient skin cleansers, which also strip the skin of its natural oils (sebum). In the case of my wife, I made especially for her an emollient cleanser (B. Kamins Bio-Maple Creamy Cleanser) that does the job nicely and helps solve her age-related dry-skin problems.

2. Exfoliate Regularly

Exfoliation, or the act of removing the skin's surface layer of dead cells, is vital for a brighter complexion and diminishing the appearance of fine lines. This skin renewal is done either once or twice a week, depending on the skin type and level of sensitivity.

There are mechanical exfoliants that require circular movements on the skin, and biological or chemical exfoliants that, once applied, are left on the skin to eat away at the dead cells. Mechanical exfoliants can differ in their degree of abrasiveness. Loofahs, synthetic scrubbing sponges, and exfoliating gloves are coarse in texture and useful for exfoliating the body. Biological or chemical exfoliants such as jojoba beads, rice beads, and finely ground nutshells can be gentle on the skin and are suitable for the face. Other ingredients such as apricot shells and pumice are much harsher and unsuitable for the face. Exfoliants come in various forms, such as scrubs, cleansers, creams, and masks.

It is important to select specific exfoliating ingredients depending on your skin type, whether dry, oily, combination, acneic, or sensitive. If the exfoliating ingredient is in a creamy base, it is usually more gentle and nourishing, and appropriate for normal to dry skin. If the ingredient is in an oil-free solution with foaming action, it is usually best for nonsensitive, oilier skin.

After exfoliating the skin, it is not uncommon to feel some transient tingling, especially after using alpha or beta hydroxy acids. It is important to rinse your skin with water to hydrate it and then super-saturate with a moisturizer to quench the new cells.

Your skin type will dictate the frequency of your exfoliation. You can exfoliate once a week if you have dry or sensitive skin, twice a week if your skin is normal, dark, oily, or acne prone. During winter months, cut back on exfoliating if your skin becomes ultradry and flaky.

If you have rosacea, exfoliation is not recommended, as the skin is already red, irritated, inflamed, and may have papules or pustules (bumps or whiteheads). Also, avoid exfoliating if you have acne with pustules. If an exfoliating ingredient breaks the thin membrane covering the pustule, bacteria can travel to other areas of the face and spread the acne. This can be extremely painful too. If you have a tendency toward acne but no pustules are present, try using either BHA (salicylic acid) or AHA (lactic acid, glycolic acid) when you exfoliate to help heal the skin.

3. Use a Healing Mask

For some people, a mask is a useful product for exfoliation or for brightening the skin. To find the mask that's right for you, follow the guidelines below:

- **For dry skin,** use a nondrying mask with a creamy consistency that contains oils, humectants, and essential fatty acids to hydrate the skin and increase cellular renewal.
- **For oily skin,** use an oil-free mask that hardens and has a tightening, oil-absorbing effect to reduce the appearance of enlarged pores.
- **For normal skin,** use a combination clay-creamy mask to absorb excess sebum, hydrate and exfoliate the skin, and help maintain healthy skin tone.

4. Use the Proper Moisturizer for Your Skin Type

We recommend moisturizing every morning and evening after you cleanse your skin. Moisturize again after using an exfoliant. Continue to moisturize throughout the day to keep your skin super-saturated.

Soak and Super-Saturate

To gain optimum benefit from your moisturizer, apply it immediately after taking a warm bath or shower. This technique, which I call "soak and super-saturate," helps to keep moisture locked in.

5. Use Beyond Botox Hydrating Tips for Areas that Need Extra Attention

- **The under-eye area.** Moisturize the under-eye area morning and night, and as needed throughout the day if this delicate skin feels dry and uncomfortable. As the thinnest skin of the body, the eye area is the first to show signs of aging. Apply under-eye cream very gently by patting it onto the skin using the ring finger. Start at the outer eye area and pat to the inner area to avoid aggravating any lines or wrinkles. It is not necessary to apply the cream directly under the lash line; rather, apply it along the orbital bone.

  Eye creams may contain antioxidants such as vitamins A and E to protect against free radicals. Other ingredients include hydrating compounds like wheat germ oil, specific ingredients for conditions such as dark under-eye circles, esculin (horse chestnut extract) for puffiness, zinc oligopeptide for wrinkles, and soy sterol for irritation. Unless specified, eye cream should not be applied to the eyelids.

- **The lips.** Regularly apply a moisturizing lip treatment that contains an SPF ingredient to protect from sun damage. Select a product that has emollients to soften lips and soothe chapped skin and dryness. We recommend the emollients squalane, carnauba wax, petrolatum, and silicone in lip products.

- **The hands.** Because the hands are regularly exposed to the sun, use a moisturizer with SPF and apply it liberally as needed. It is best to apply the moisturizer to the backs of the hands first (instead of the palms), since dryness is more pronounced on the backs of the hands. Hand creams have emollients that moisturize and protect against the drying effect of soaps and detergents.

- **The feet and heels.** The feet and heels are especially prone to thickened skin (hyperkeratinization), calluses, skin cracking, itchiness, and irritation. Treatments include ingredients that will soothe, smooth, soften, relieve irritation, and moisturize. Foot creams usually have peppermint oil, menthol, menthyl lactate, or a combination of these, since these ingredients are cooling and refreshing. AHAs such as glycolic acid help to smooth skin and exfoliate dead cells, stimulating new, softer and healthier skin.
- **The neck.** Most women forget to moisturize the neck in their daily skin care regimen. Creams applied to this area should be moisturizing, firming, occlusive, and film forming.
- **The elbows.** The texture of the elbows tends to be rough, uneven, and often dry. Just as with feet and heels, AHAs such as glycolic acid help to smooth elbow skin and exfoliate dead cells while stimulating new skin. Emollients also help soften skin.

Beyond Botox Recommendations for Super-Saturate

1. Follow a consistent regimen for sexy, ageless skin.

2. Exfoliate regularly.

3. Try a healing mask.

4. Use the proper moisturizer for your skin type.

5. Use Beyond Botox hydrating tips for sensitive areas.

Chapter 9

Step #6: Pamper

Become Spa Savvy for Wellness and Balance

Since ancient Roman soldiers in a small Belgian village called Spa discovered the soothing effects that hot mineral springs had on their aching bodies, spas have been associated with healing. Around the turn of the twentieth century, French physicians would send patients to spas to treat exhaustion or achy muscles or joints. Over time, spas developed into the consummate symbol of balance, wellness, and luxury.

Today, spas continue to offer refreshment and relief from the everyday rigors of life. While still focused on wellness, most spas are affordable and provide an extensive menu of healing treatments that are well suited for every woman — no matter what her age, specific needs, or time constraints. These often-lavish havens offer consolation for today's woman who desperately needs time apart from her frenzied routine to focus on herself and become centered once again.

In Steps 1 through 5, I presented a plan to create sexy, ageless skin by making simple lifestyle changes. In Step 6, I want to show you how to find a sense of serenity and balance in your life with a spa experience — by spending time at a day spa periodically, taking your vacation at a resort spa, or creating your own soothing spa experience in the privacy of your home.

Indulgence as Insurance for Health and Beauty

Ask any health care professional how to age well, and most will say that the key to maintaining wellness and youthfulness is to take personal responsibility for yourself each day. This does not mean memorizing your doctor's phone number so you can quickly get the latest medication to "cure" what ails you. As a pharmaceutical chemist, I'll be the first to tell you that taking medications needlessly can cause more health problems than not. Rather, taking responsibility for yourself means making the right lifestyle choices each day — getting proper nutrients in your daily diet, exercising moderately, finding your sleep zone, and coping positively with the stress in your life.

But if you are time crunched yet in desperate need of solace from the frantic pace of life, I want you to consider taking time out regularly to pamper yourself. Whether fully immersed in career, family, or community activities, most women traditionally put everyone else ahead of themselves when it comes to personal wellness and balance. However, when you take care of yourself — your mind, body, *and* spirit — you have a powerful weapon against life's stressors.

Though we all strive for balance in our lives, sometimes it's hard to stay on top of our health with all the distractions fighting for our time and attention. That's when you need to think about imposing pampering upon yourself. Not only will you feel healthier if you take regular time to pamper yourself, you'll feel and look younger too.

Unlike conventional health care that aims to treat physical or emotional symptoms, the spa philosophy embraces the concept of wholeness and offers services that function to meld the mind, body, and spirit. These natural therapies are based on the science behind psychoneuroimmunology, or the premise that mental or emotional processes (the mind) affect physiologic function (the body). Experts in the field of psychoneuroimmunology link 90 to 95 percent of all health problems to the influence of emotions. They maintain that an optimistic outlook, such as a feeling of control, may in some way protect against disease or illness and act as a valuable complement to conventional medical care.

Those on the cutting edge of mind-body therapies believe that many influences are at work in each of us that either keep us well or cause us to get sick. For example, scientific evidence suggests that factors such as stress, negative feelings, and lack of social support can influence immune status and function, as well as speed disease onset and progression. Although still early in its development, research suggests that psychological factors may play a role in autoimmune diseases such as allergies, asthma, arthritis, and multiple sclerosis, as well as serious chronic illnesses like cardiovascular disease and cancer.

Pampering Yourself for Sexy, Ageless Skin

Diana's story reveals what most women experience their first time at a spa:

> When I turned fifty last year, some colleagues at the middle school where I teach treated me to a morning of pampering at a nearby day spa. Having never been to a spa before, I always thought it was for women who simply had too much time on their hands. Was I wrong!
>
> When I arrived, I was given a luxurious white terry cloth robe and warm booties to wear and was taken into a small room for a sea salt treatment. The spa technician rubbed a luxurious blend of sea salts and oils all over my body, massaging it gently into my skin. Then she washed the salt scrub off with a misting spray and applied another gentle moisturizer until my skin was incredibly smooth and shiny.
>
> I then had a manicure and pedicure. After a therapeutic hand and foot soak, the technician softened and smoothed my cuticles and shaped my nails. She used warm essential oil–infused compresses to cleanse my skin, and massaged my feet and calves with this delightful, tingly moisturizer. I then placed my feet and hands in plastic bags filled with warm paraffin wax. After about fifteen minutes, the technician peeled the wax off and rinsed the skin. I could not believe how soft my skin was after the wax treatment, and those little aches and pains in my fingers were gone completely. It made me think about how much I rely on my hands and feet yet how little I really pamper them.
>
> Next I received a facial treatment and upper-shoulder and décolleté massage by the aesthetician, a licensed cosmetologist. As she gently massaged my face with a hydrating and revitalizing treatment, she gave me some suggestions

on caring for my skin and even recommended several anti-aging skin care products.

A massage therapist (also licensed) then led me into a small candlelit room where soft music was playing. For about thirty minutes, she massaged my entire back, using incredibly light and rhythmic strokes to relieve the stress and tension in my muscles. When she told me the massage was over, I didn't want to get up. I was relaxed and so contented.

If you, like Diana, have never been to a spa before, it can seem overwhelming trying to decide which spa experience is best — much less feeling bold enough to make an appointment. Perhaps this virtual tour of the various types of spas will help you understand some of the spa terminology and feel more comfortable about making an appointment to take advantage of spa pampering and mind-body rejuvenation.

Day Spas

If you want to have a facial or a manicure and pedicure, you should visit a day spa, a full-service spa available in most large cities. Treatments at day spas include hour-long massages to half-day or full-day spa packages that include manicures, pedicures, skin conditioning, facials, exfoliation, massage, wraps and packs, hair removal, fitness classes, hydrotherapy, and much more.

A facial at a day spa can help regenerate the skin, boost cell energy, and reverse the natural aging process. The spa's aesthetician, a specially trained and licensed cosmetologist, can evaluate your skin and then recommend special cosmeceuticals or other spa therapies that might help to reverse some of the visible signs of aging and revitalize pasty, ultradry, or oily skin.

Medical Spas

If you want more than a rejuvenating facial or healing massage, you might consider a medical spa, or medi-spa, a facility whose medical program is run under the strict supervision of a licensed health care professional, usually a dermatologist or plastic surgeon. Medical spas blend spa services with conventional and alternative healing therapies, and their numbers are on the rise: nationally, medical spas have increased from 250 to 1,250 in the past five years.

Medical spas offer facials, massages, and body treatments, along with more invasive skin therapies like laser treatments and collagen injections. Many offer holistic healing practices such as acupuncture and biofeedback. Some spas provide health testing such as bone density scans, lipid analysis, and electrocardiograms. The physician on staff at the medical spa can help evaluate and treat lifestyle problems such as chronic stress, headaches, sleep problems, weight management, and muscle or joint discomfort.

Resort Spas

Resort spas are located within a resort or hotel and provide professionally administered spa services, fitness and wellness components, and spa cuisine. The resort spa provides myriad therapeutic and relaxing services such as massage, facials, manicures and pedicures, and exfoliations, along with elegant dining experiences and even tours of local surroundings. Many resort spas have state-of-the-art fitness centers to help clients sculpt their bodies, lose weight, or get back in shape using weight-training machines, treadmills, stair-climbers, elliptical trainers, bikes, swimming pools, and rowing machines, among other things. Resort spas have packages for singles, couples, and even families.

What's an Aesthetician?

An aesthetician is someone who has specific training in skin care and has completed all the requirements of the state in which he or she practices. This licensed cosmetologist performs facials as well as other aesthetic spa services such as nail care, makeup application, hair removal, hair care, and certain body treatments. To ensure that an aesthetician is knowledgeable, ask about specific training and certification. For more information about your state's requirements, go to http://www.dermalinstitute.com/e_library/useful_links_StateBoards.asp.

What's a Spa Facial?

No matter how well you take care of your skin at home, there are always benefits to receiving a facial at a professional spa. Apart from the standard cleansing and exfoliation, a spa facial includes a relaxing massage of the face, neck, head, and shoulders in a pleasant, calming, stress-free environment. If requested, specialized procedures such as extractions (cleaning the pores) and micro-exfoliations can also be included, as well as facial-hair removal. Plus, having someone pamper you for a few hours is indulgent fun!

Ancient Therapies to New Age Trends

Most spas offer far more than facials, exfoliations, and skin consultations. Along with the various types of bodywork and massage discussed in Step 4, Relax (page 116), there are licensed professionals who use ancient healing modalities like acupuncture, acupressure, shiatsu, and Ayurvedic body massage, among other natural therapies to relieve stress and restore health.

Acupuncture Boosts Endorphins

Yes, this is the treatment with the needles. And no, it doesn't hurt! Let's discuss this a bit so you can learn how acupuncture works and why it is wonderfully effective for many people.

Not only does acupuncture provide pain relief and improve function for individuals with problems such as osteoarthritis (the "wear and tear" arthritis), but many health care professionals confirm that acupuncture is an effective complement to standard medical treatment for some problems. In the field of dermatology, acupuncture has been reported to be beneficial for the treatment of acne, psoriasis, atopic dermatitis, and hives, among other skin problems associated with stress.

In applying this healing art, a trained practitioner inserts one or more dry needles into the skin and underlying tissues at specific points on the body. The stimulation of these acupuncture points with the needles produces rhythmic discharges in nerve fibers, causing the release of endorphins, the "feel good" hormones that can help you relax and feel positive. There is scientific evidence that acupuncture may positively change the way the brain interprets pain and other external sensations, which may give relief for many chronic illnesses.

If you want to try acupuncture, make sure you select a licensed acupuncturist with vast experience who uses only disposable needles. At this time, there are more than 6,500 certified and licensed practitioners in the United States, and more than 3,000 of these are conventional medical doctors. For recommendations, you can write or call the American Academy of Medical Acupuncture (AAMA) or check out their Web site at www.medicalacupuncture.org.

Does Acupuncture Really Work?

According to a National Institutes of Health (NIH) consensus panel of scientists, researchers, and practitioners, the answer is yes. They found that acupuncture may be useful by itself or when combined with conventional therapies to treat addiction, headaches, menstrual cramps, tennis elbow, fibromyalgia, myofascial pain, osteoarthritis, lower-back pain, carpal tunnel syndrome, and asthma and to assist in stroke rehabilitation.

Acupressure Reduces Tension

Unlike its similarly named relative, acupressure, another form of Chinese healing, uses *touch* instead of needles to unblock Chi (the flow of energy throughout the body) and allow the meridians or pathways of energy to flow smoothly. For example, pressing a specific acupressure point on the wrist (called the P6, or Neiguan, point) has been found to be effective for some types of motion sickness.

With acupressure, the practitioner uses the fingers to press key points on the surface of the skin to stimulate the body's natural self-curative abilities. Pressure is applied gently initially but then increases to the point where a strong sensation is felt. Using acupressure regularly helps to trigger the relaxation response, the physiological state that is characterized by a feeling of warmth and quiet mental alertness. You may also experience less muscle tension and reduced pain in the muscles and joints.

Shiatsu Increases Relaxation

Another popular spa therapy is shiatsu, an ancient Japanese healing art that is also based upon the concept of Chi. The shiatsu practitioner uses his or her hands, elbows, knees, and even feet to press various points along twelve meridians, or pathways, in the body in order to balance energy. The pressure is held for several seconds and is repeated several times. It is thought that this pressure helps stimulate the body's endorphins to produce a tranquilizing effect, or it may help by loosening up muscles and improving blood circulation. With shiatsu, the practitioner may also use pulling and pushing strokes, tapping, rubbing, and squeezing to influence the body's tissues.

Ayurvedic Massage

Ayurvedic massage, body massage with oil and spices, is an ancient therapy that focuses on relaxation and the prevention of disease. It is another spa favorite used for stress-related illnesses, to reverse the damage from negative lifestyle habits, and to maintain balance in the body. According to this five-thousand-year-old traditional Indian system of medicine, health is the state of balance and disease is the state of imbalance. Its premise is that there are three physiological forces called *doshas* (*vata, pitta,* and *kapha*). All of us are made of a combination of *doshas* that give us a particular metabolic type yet have one *dosha* that dominates. *Vata* people are thin and energetic, *pittas* are hot tempered, and *kaphas* are slow and solid.

Ayurvedic massage is said to unblock invisible *marma* points through which energy flows. When this energy is freed, your body heals itself. Abhayanga massage (four-handed, or dual, massage) is offered at many spas throughout the world today. Using special herbal oil chosen for your particular *dosha*, two therapists massage you at the same time. This intense touch therapy is followed by an energetic rubdown with a coarse towel.

Reflexology Increases Relaxation

Reflexology, or zone therapy, is a healing art based on the theory that there are reflex areas, or specific points, in the feet and hands that correspond to all the glands and organs in the body. The term *reflex* refers to the fact that these points are responsive to stimulus.

As with acupuncture and other touch modalities, reflexology is based on the belief that nerve pathways exist throughout the body. When any of these pathways is blocked, the body experiences discomfort or "disease." Reflexology is thought to revive this energy flow and bring the body back into homeostasis, or a state of balance.

There are not numerous clinical trials to support this healing art, but one randomized, controlled study from the School of Nursing at East Carolina University in Greenville, North Carolina, found that twenty-three patients with breast or lung cancer experienced improvement in anxiety and pain when treated with foot reflexology.

Reflex Points and Corresponding Body Zones

Reflex Point	Corresponding Body Zone
Metatarsal (ball of the foot)	Chest, lungs, and shoulder area
Toes	Head and neck
Upper arch	Diaphragm, upper abdominal organs
Lower arch	Pelvic and lower abdominal organs
Heel	Pelvic and sciatic nerve
Outer foot	Arm, shoulder, hip, leg, knee, and lower back
Inner foot	Spine
Ankle area	Reproductive organs and pelvic region

Reiki Improves Emotional Health

Reiki, the Japanese word for "universal life force energy," is an ancient energy-channeling technique that releases Chi that is blocked in the body. Many of today's day spas, medical spas, and resort spas offer Reiki to patrons who want to improve physical and emotional health and reduce stress.

With Reiki, the practitioner places her or his hands on or near the client's body in a series of positions. Each position, whether on the hands, feet, shoulders, or other area, is held for three to ten minutes depending on how much Reiki the client needs. The entire treatment usually lasts between forty and ninety minutes. This subtle form of healing may be done through clothing and without any physical contact between the practitioner and client.

If used effectively, Reiki aids in boosting energy, healing, and mental clarity, and decreases pain. Stress reduction with some improvement in one's physical and psychological condition are what most experience.

Make a Spa Heating Pad

Make a cozy heat wrap: Fill a heavy sock with whole flaxseed. Sew or tie the end. Or sew two washcloths or small fingertip towels together to make a heating pad. Fill the cloth with flaxseed and sew it closed. To use, place the heat wrap or pad in the microwave, along with a cup of water, for one to two minutes and heat until warm. (Make sure the microwave rotates the pad or the seed can burn.)

Shaping Up at the Spa

Along with the exotic healing arts, larger spas offer body conditioning with Pilates, yoga, and tai chi. Let's look at these popular spa activities.

Pilates Improves Body Alignment

Devised by Joseph Pilates, a German gymnast and boxer, in the early part of the twentieth century, Pilates is based on the concept of strengthening the body's "powerhouse" — the corset of muscles around the pelvis and lower abdomen. Pilates believed that when these muscles are under strain, other joints and muscles will be stressed as well. Today, this system of strengthening and stretching exercises focusing on the "core" has become extremely popular, with more than five hundred Pilates studios across the nation.

Yoga Reduces Tension

Yoga is an ancient form of exercise that has also grown enormously in popularity in the past decade. You can find a yoga class in almost any town, and guided DVDs, videocassettes, and CDs abound. Yoga can reduce stress and relieve muscular tension or pain by increasing the body's flexibility and strength. Practicing yoga when you're feeling tense or anxious may help to reduce stress and the risk of injury. With any type of yoga, you may find great benefit from the physical postures (asanas) to alleviate aches and pains, concentration exercises (dharana) to overcome dwelling on your pain problem, and meditation (dhyana) to help you focus on the present instead of ruminating about worries.

Tai Chi Increases Balance and Flexibility

Tai chi uses a series of flowing, graceful movements that develop muscular strength without straining the joints. Not only does tai chi provide a good workout, it also helps to increase balance and flexibility while preventing falls and injury. Those who practice tai chi claim to bend easier and to be better able to do daily tasks at home and work.

Spa Hydrotherapy

The use of hydrotherapy goes back to ancient Greece, where all forms of water — from ice to steam — were used to promote healing and well-being. Today's spas use hydrotherapy as a method of stimulating the client's own healing force. For instance, cold compresses are placed on the skin to reduce inflammation by constricting blood vessels, helping to control minor internal bleeding. Conversely, warm, moist compresses are placed on the skin to dilate blood vessels, which in turn lowers blood pressure, increasing the flow of blood, with its oxygen and nutrients, and speeding the elimination of toxins.

Many spa patrons find long-lasting relief with balneotherapy, or the use of hot baths or Jacuzzis to alleviate tension and stress. This centuries-old therapy helps to increase muscle relaxation, boost blood supply to the site, and relieve muscle rigidity and spasms.

Epsom salts or bicarbonate of soda can be added to therapeutic warm baths to assist in detoxification.

Use a Jacuzzi for Deep Sleep

Try using a Jacuzzi an hour or two before bedtime. The soothing hot water will warm your skin, relax muscle tension, and prepare your body for deep, restorative "beauty" sleep. Caution: avoid hot Jacuzzis if you have diabetes, high blood pressure, cardiovascular disease, or are pregnant.

Preparing for Your Spa Experience

All spas specialize in wellness. That said, when selecting which spa you want to enjoy, you must decide what it is you want.

• Do you want a facial or a massage? A day spa close to your home or work will offer a variety of facials and massages, allowing you to use these services regularly for stress reduction and anti-aging.

• Do you want a professional skin assessment and more invasive therapies, such as microdermabrasion or more aggressive chemical peels? Then a medi-spa, or medical spa, is the one you would select.

• Do you want to meet friends for a weeklong spa excursion or take your children or grandchildren with you while you enjoy spa amenities? In this case, a resort or destination spa would best suit your needs.

It is important to identify what it is that you want to accomplish with a spa and then select the one that enables you to concentrate on your goals, whether skin care, fitness, stress management, nutrition, pain or tension relief, or all-out pampering.

All spas offer a menu of services that briefly describes the treatments or activities, the therapeutic value, the time allotted, and the cost. While you can make online reservations for larger spas, it is wise to talk to the reservation–front desk staff. It is helpful to have a list of questions written down that you want to ask this person. For example, consider the following:

1. What is the cancellation policy?

2. Are the therapists male or female? (You should always specify your preference ahead of time.)

3. Is there a specific dress code?

4. For day spa packages, are substitutions of therapies allowed other than what they have advertised? (Some women prefer to select their own options instead of taking a package.)

5. Are there any counterindications to treatments such as deep-tissue massage or a sauna if a medical condition exists?

6. Are there any specials currently available?

When making the reservation, be sure to state your preference for a male or female therapist. As an example, for a deep-tissue massage or sports massage to help ease pain in a strained muscle, male massage therapists are more sought after, since they are generally stronger. If you are uncomfortable with a male massage therapist, make sure you convey this to the reception staff. Also, ask about the spa's cancellation policy. Because credit card numbers are usually required to guarantee bookings, more spas are charging no-show or late fees.

The reception staff will explain treatments of interest and give brief descriptions of services offered. For example, if you want a body wrap that will help ease sore muscles or a deep-muscle massage that will promote relaxation and ease pain, the reception staff will let you know which modalities are best. There is the possibility of add-ons during the treatment, which may be obtained à la carte, meaning you can select optional therapies from a listing.

To find out if the spa is hygienic, go straight to the management and ask the following:

1. What do you use to disinfect instruments if someone has fungus on nails?

2. Do you have an autoclave or pressurized device that heats water above the boiling point in order to kill bacteria?

3. Are sheets changed after each treatment?

Spas should use an antibacterial cleanser as well as a sterilizer that reaches high temperatures to kill bacteria on any spa item that is used by clients. Disinfection with rubbing alcohol is not adequate!

Spa Attire

Most of the time, *you* decide what you will or will not wear at a spa, depending on the type of treatment or activity. If you're not sure what is standard, feel free to ask the receptionist when booking your appointment or at the front desk when you check in. There are no stupid questions at a spa! Believe me, they've heard them all, and they shouldn't laugh at any question or concern you bring up. Remember: their number one job is to make you feel comfortable.

If a gown or robe is required for bodywork or massage, the therapist will only expose the portion of the body that is being treated at the time. Sometimes a swimsuit may be appropriate if the treatment includes water.

If you are taking a yoga or tai chi class, it is best to wear loose pants and a shirt. If you are receiving more than one treatment or if you are at a resort-destination spa, the spa's management often prefers to have clients sport bathrobes and slippers to minimize changing times between treatments and to ensure the clients' comfort and overall positive experience.

Calculating Gratuities

There is no one standard for tipping. Some spas have specific tipping policies for their facility and can explain the policy when you pay your bill. Some spas automatically include the tip in the bill as a service charge. A general guideline for gratuities is between 15 and 20 percent of the treatment cost.

Finding the Best Spas

Check out spa associations, publications, and Web sites that can help with finding a reputable spa. Many of these have lists of spa members that have undergone inspection and meet strict standards. For more information about the spa industry, go to www.experienceispa.com, which is the site of the International Spa Association (ISPA), www.dayspaassociation.com, and www.spafinder.com.

Putting the Program into Action

Pamper for Sexy, Ageless Skin

Become Spa Savvy for Wellness and Balance

1. Start Your Spa Experience

Spas offer so many healing therapies that it would be impossible to describe all of them. Use the following list to review popular spa offerings, and checkmark the treatments that you might enjoy.

Menu of Treatments and Activities

____Facial
____Rosacea facial
____Scalp and/or facial massage
____Makeover
____Manicure/pedicure
____Paraffin wax treatment
____Waxing
____Massage
____Cellulite treatment
____Mud bath
____Herbal wrap
____Sea salt scrub
____Seaweed wrap
____Hydrotherapy
____Acupuncture
____Acupressure
____Shiatsu
____Reflexology
____Reiki
____Fitness class
____Pilates
____Yoga
____Tai chi

____Swimming

____Sauna

It is best to arrive about fifteen minutes before your first appointment in order to go over the scheduled appointments and complete a health form. At medical or destination spas, a consultation with a wellness director or medical personnel is frequently booked before receiving any treatments. Once checked in, at many spas, clients are taken on a tour to familiarize them with the relaxation area and other amenities offered, such as weight room, fitness center, pool, and sauna. Lockers are usually available in changing rooms to store personal items.

2. Bring the Spa Experience Home

Along with the fabulous skin- and body-rejuvenation therapies, many women seek the spa experience as an escape from the rigors of daily life. However, when spa time is hard to come by, you can easily create your own luxury spa in the privacy of your home. Here are some suggestions:

- **Dress for relaxation.** Purchase a terry cloth robe strictly to use for your home spa experience. Keep this in your bathroom so you can easily change from street clothes into the loose-fitting robe.
- **Create a spa ambience.** You may have experienced how favorite fragrances can brighten your mood or even relax you when you are stressed. For instance, lavender and spiced apples are thought to activate the alpha wave activity in the back of the brain, which leads to relaxation. Jasmine and lemon are used to increase beta wave activity in the front of the brain, which is associated with alertness. Researchers have found that when you inhale aromatic molecules, they bind to receptors and build electrical impulses that move up the olfactory nerves to the brain. The ultimate target is the limbic system, where your emotions and memory are processed.

If you enjoy fragrances, fill your bathroom with aromatherapy candles with relaxing fragrances like lavender, chamomile, sandalwood, orange blossom, spiced apple, and vanilla. If fragrances bother you, use unscented candles for mood lighting alone.

- **Add a plant or two.** The bathroom, with its high humidity, is the perfect environment for houseplants. Select plants that need low to moderate light.
- **Enjoy music therapy.** Bring a portable CD player with speakers into the bathroom and enjoy soft, soothing music as you seek to create a tranquil, spa-like environment.
- **Visualize calmness.** Gather framed photographs of your favorite vacation destinations, such as an ocean sunset or a mountain waterfall, and place these on your bathroom vanity. Try to visualize the tranquillity you felt at each locale using the steps described on page 125.
- **Taste healing foods.** Enjoy a cool glass of Green Tea Skin Saver (page 74) or room temperature red wine during your bath and benefit from their supernutrients for your skin. (Always use plastic — not glass — in the bathroom to prevent accidents.)
- **Soak and super-saturate.** Soak at least fifteen minutes in a warm bath to take advantage of the moist heat on tired skin and sore muscles and joints. You can add two cups of Epsom salts to boost the healing effect of the bath.

  During your bath, spend time exfoliating by gently rubbing your skin with a washcloth, soft sponge, or loofah to remove dead cells. A razor is a good exfoliant for your legs.

  After your bath, stand on a dry towel and saturate your skin with pure mineral oil or your favorite moisturizer to keep it hydrated. Avoid getting the oil on your face or in your eyes. After your skin is well hydrated, pat yourself dry with a soft towel.

- **Focus on your face.** While pores are open after the bath, exfoliate your face, pluck your eyebrows, and notice any skin changes. You can gently boost skin circulation by applying a moisturizer to your fingertips and then massaging it on your face. Review the charts in Step 5, Super-Saturate to find the therapies suited to your skin type.
- **Focus on your hands.** Rub your favorite moisturizer on your hands and cuticles and massage them gently. While doing so, try a spa hand massage that focuses on the pressure points

that relieve mental tension. Take your right thumb and press it firmly into the soft tissue area between your left thumb and forefinger, breathing slowly while doing so. Switch hands and do the same for your right hand.

Beyond Botox Recommendations for Pamper

1. Start your spa experience at a day spa, medical spa, or resort spa.

2. Bring the spa experience home.

Chapter 10

Step #7: Radiate

Combat Specific Skin Problems . . . at Any Age

When I was a boy of eight or nine, I met for the first time my two uncles who had immigrated to Canada from Poland and Austria. As I stared up at these towering men, I wondered if I would ever look like them — with their extremely fair complexions, blond hair, blue eyes, and very red faces. As an adult I realized that my uncles actually had a skin condition called rosacea, which is characterized by a ruddy complexion, but I only discovered this when I myself was diagnosed with the same condition about forty years later.

What do *you* see when you look into the mirror each morning? Perhaps you notice dark under-eye circles or crow's-feet just like your mother's and grandmother's. Or maybe you have fair, delicate skin that burns easily like your sister or an aunt. It is not uncommon to come across a strong genetic component with many skin problems. For instance, if your mother had dry, scaly skin and fine lines and wrinkles at a young age, the chances are great that you and your siblings might experience the same. Likewise, if oily skin with blemishes runs in your family, the chance that you will have to deal with this problem is greatly increased. Even some types of skin cancer have a genetic link, particularly melanoma.

But despite our predispositions to certain skin conditions, there is good news: we can outsmart our genes and maintain beautiful skin. I believe that optimal skin appearance comes from protecting and nourishing the skin as much as possible — from the inside, as we discussed in the previous six strategies, and from the outside, as this last strategy introduces. Every woman can prevent those skin conditions over which she has control and seek an accurate diagnosis and effective treatment in the earliest stages of development of a new skin problem, when targeted therapies are most effective. No woman needs to have prematurely "old-looking" skin; by taking care of skin problems early, before they result in permanent scarring or premature aging, you can keep your skin healthy for years to come. By understanding the treatments available, you can take an active role in maintaining an ageless complexion.

In this chapter, I'll take a look at some of the most common complaints I hear about from clients — problems like rosacea, adult acne, and crow's-feet — and show you how to be proactive about combating them and keeping your skin vibrant, healthy, and beautiful.

Common Skin Conditions at Any Age

Where do you turn when your skin problems flare? Over the past decade, my son and business partner, Howard, has traveled the globe, meeting with professionals at thousands of resort and destination spas, day spas, and medi-spas nationally and internationally. It distresses him greatly when aestheticians share horror stories of clients who have tried to camouflage serious skin problems such as acne or rosacea, using layer after layer of cover cream, powder, or thick, oily foundation to hide the reddened complexion, pimples, cysts, and irritated skin. The trouble with this "self-care" approach, as I see it, is that most of the time these women are simply putting a Band-Aid on the problem instead of treating the actual cause. And women who try to disguise a skin condition instead of seeking proper treatment usually end up with far greater problems, including ultradry or oily skin, flaky skin, blemishes, itchy rashes, uneven skin tone, drab or older-looking skin, and worsened acne or rosacea conditions.

The reality is that many physicians push aside cosmetic concern when dealing with patients. After all, the number one killer of women is cardiovascular disease, not wrinkled skin. Nonetheless, with a life expectancy of about 81 years, a fifty-one-year-old woman can expect to live more than one-third of her life after menopause. My wife is a perfect example of an active, vibrant, intelligent woman who has greatly benefited from my responsible, noninvasive skin care regimen. I've also worked on several other skin conditions that usually fall under the radar for popularity. These include smoker's skin, diabetic skin, acne-rosacea, and sensitive skin, which together affect millions of people.

In this last step, Radiate, I have identified the most common skin problems women have in various stages in the life cycle. My definitions of the different life cycle stages — and the skin issues that come with them — are purposefully broad. For example, some of these skin problems (such as acne) can occur at various times throughout one's life. But no matter when they occur, these are problems that women treat — and mistreat — with an arsenal of remedies and over-the-counter and prescription therapies. I'll try to help you find the therapy that is right for you.

Find the optimal approach for your individual situation and decide which of these skin problems should send you to the doctor immediately, and which ones you can self-treat and monitor with the remedies listed. Even if these common conditions do not affect you, following the basic prevention strategies provided may still improve your overall skin health.

Skin Concerns for the Twenties

Acne

Freckles

Rosacea

Pregnancy mask (melasma)

Moles (nevi)

Skin Concerns for the Thirties

Fine lines and wrinkles

Under-eye circles

Skin tags (acrochordon)

Décolleté health

Skin Concerns for the Forties

Perimenopausal skin

Liver spots (solar lentigo)

Crow's-feet

Eczema
Lip lines

Skin Concerns for the Fifties and Beyond

Menopausal skin
Spider veins (telangiectasia)
Skin cancer (carcinoma)
Diabetes and skin problems
Postmenopausal skin

Skin Concerns for the Twenties

Most women in their early twenties have few fine lines and wrinkles because the skin functions optimally, holding in the necessary moisture and stretching to keep the outward surface taut and smooth. Fibers called elastin give the skin an elastic quality, locking in moisture and allowing the skin to stretch. Collagen, the major structural protein in the dermis, also plays a key role in preventing wrinkles by supporting the epidermis, or outer layer of skin.

At this age, many women still experience pimples or acne. While the outbreak of pimples may be acute (short-term and appearing suddenly) and coincide with the menstrual cycle or stress, many women in their twenties suffer with chronic (long-term, or persistent) acne, which can be difficult to treat if not managed properly.

As women approach thirty, they begin to see the start of wrinkling and blotchiness as a direct result of accumulated sun exposure during childhood and adolescence. Women in their twenties should use an appropriate emollient moisturizer around the eye area, an oil-free sunscreen, and an antioxidant daily moisturizer under their makeup. If you are struggling with acne, try a cleanser that has ingredients such as salicylic acid, lactic acid, and/or glycolic acid.

Acne

What is it? Acne is an inflammatory skin problem, typically appearing on the face, scalp, neck, shoulders, chest, and back, and characterized by tender pimples, irritated skin, and clogged pores. There is a genetic link to acne, and it is also related to an increase in hormones called androgens (male sex hormones), which increase during puberty and cause the sebaceous glands to enlarge and produce more sebum. But acne is not just for kids and young adults. More than 40 million Americans suffer with acne, as the skin disease continues into adulthood, even into the thirties and forties, affecting both men and women. Acne can cause emotional anguish and possibly pitting and scarring of the skin, but if you treat the condition quickly, it is rarely serious.

What causes it? Hormonal changes appear to stimulate the oil-producing (sebaceous) skin glands and trigger acne. Other hormonal changes, including pregnancy, menstrual periods, and the use of birth control pills, can also aggravate acne. External triggers such as cosmetics, facial creams, hair dyes, and greasy cosmetic and hair ointments may lead to the development of acne or exacerbate existing acne. Clothing that rubs the skin may also worsen the disorder, as can heavy sweating and humid climates. Even stress is a known trigger. If effective prevention and treatment measures are started early, you can keep acne under control.

Who's at risk? Acne is the most common skin condition in the United States. About 85 percent of the adolescent population experiences acne at some time. Acne affects 8 percent of adults ages twenty-five to thirty-four and 3 percent of adults thirty-five to forty-four.

Signs and symptoms: Acne usually affects those areas of the body with the greatest number of sebaceous glands (the neck, face, chest, upper back, and upper arms). Acne starts when blocked pores on the skin produce whiteheads. If the pores stay open and trap dirt, the plugs may darken, causing blackheads. When the blocked pores become infected or inflamed, it causes pimples, or raised red spots with white centers. Cysts form when blockage and inflammation deep inside hair follicles produce lumps beneath the surface of the skin.

Prevention and treatment: Acne treatments work by reducing oil production, speeding up skin cell turnover, fighting bacterial infection, or doing all three. Start by washing problem areas with a gentle cleanser and warm water two to three times a day. Avoid overwashing, as this causes further skin irritation.

Over-the-counter ingredients that can help to resolve acne pimples include benzoyl peroxide, salicylic acid, resorcinol, sodium thiosulfate, and sulfur. Avoid consuming alcohol, caffeine, hydrogenated oils, and fried food. While these do not cause acne, they may work to trigger or worsen it. There are also some studies indicating that natural hormones and bioactive molecules in milk and dairy products may exacerbate acne.

To stop acne outbreaks, researchers believe that it's important to get in control of stressful situations, as stress wreaks havoc with hormones, which may be related to acne outbreaks. You may recall from the discussion on stress the Stanford University study that found that as college students' stress levels increased, so did the severity of their acne.

Topical preparations such as retinoids (medications derived from vitamin A), azelaic acid, lactic acid, glycolic acid, salicylic acid, and benzoyl peroxide are frequently prescribed for acne. Benzoyl peroxide reduces oil production and has antibacterial properties, but it can leave the skin dry and flaky if precautions are not taken. Resorcinol, salicylic acid, and sulfur, as well as prescription retinoids, have been shown to effectively reduce blackheads, whiteheads, and the inflamed acne nodules. When there are large cysts on the upper parts of the body and on the face, these topical treatments may be combined with a topical antibiotic.

For tough cases of acne, antibiotics (oral and topical) are often used. Some antibiotics, including erythromycin, clindamycin, and tetracycline, have both antibacterial and anti-inflammatory properties and are often prescribed for daily use over a period of time (usually four to six months). Because antibiotic resistance is an increasing problem among those with acne, talk to your doctor about the course of treatment. Many physicians prescribe antibiotics only when they are necessary and make the treatment course short.

Other agents (oral medications and topical ointments) may be used with the antibiotic. Because acne is androgen dependent, if treatment fails after three to six months and the large cysts continue, a doctor may prescribe an oral contraceptive or antiandrogen for females. Oral isotretinoin (Accutane), a prescription, may also be given by a doctor if the acne involves numerous large cysts on the face, neck, and upper trunk with severe scarring. This medication is not to be used by pregnant women or women who might become pregnant, as it is associated with fetal malformations.

When to call the doctor: Although acne is not a serious medical condition, it can result in permanent scarring and pitting of the skin. Seek treatment from a dermatologist for persistent pimples or inflamed cysts to avoid scarring or other damage. If acne or the scars it has left are affecting your social relationships or self-esteem, you may want to see a dermatologist to find out if your acne can be controlled or the scars diminished. In rare cases, a sudden onset of severe acne in an older adult may signal an underlying disease. If acne strikes suddenly or without explanation in later years, see your doctor.

A Pimple or Acne?

Everyone is at risk for developing pimples. This common skin condition does not necessarily mean a flare-up of acne. Rather, pimples can result from skin infections, allergies, or even clothing rubbing on the skin. Pimple problems can be broken down into three categories: acne vulgaris, acne rosacea, and perioral dermatitis. Each category is different, as is the treatment.

Freckles

Freckles, or ephelides, are red or light brown small macules (skin spots) that darken upon exposure to sun and fade during the winter months. There may be few freckles or many, and they are usually found on the face, arms, and back. If you have freckles, always wear sunblock to prevent darkening of the ephelides. You might also try an over-the-counter treatment that contains ingredients such as hydroquinone, vitamin C ester, kojic acid, and alpha hydroxy acids (AHAs).

Rosacea

What is it? Rosacea is an acne-like skin condition that affects more than 14 million Americans, usually between the ages of twenty-five and sixty. It is characterized by redness in the central part of the face, including the nose, cheeks, eyelids, and forehead. While many skin conditions are curable, rosacea is not. It is a chronic (long-term) disorder that is characterized by periods of exacerbation (flares) and remission. The goal of treatment with rosacea is control of symptoms rather than curing the disease itself. In the most serious cases, patients suffer from large disfiguring bumps on the face, dark ruddy skin, and serious eye problems.

What causes it? The exact cause of rosacea is unknown, although there are various theories. Some scientists believe the rather disturbing theory that hair follicle mites exacerbate the inflammatory reaction. Another theory is that rosacea is caused by a generalized disorder of the blood vessels, which might explain the tendency of those with rosacea to flush easily. Still another possibility is that bacteria may be involved, causing an infection in the skin. Again, these are theories and thus far none has been proven.

Who's at risk? Rosacea commonly occurs in individuals who have very fair complexions and light eye and hair color. There is evidence that those people with a Celtic or northern European heritage are more likely to get rosacea, as are individuals who experience frequent flushing or blushing. Rosacea also has a strong genetic component and tends to run in families. In one survey taken by the National Rosacea Society, 40 percent of rosacea patients questioned responded that they had a relative with similar skin symptoms. Sometimes topical corticosteroids used for rashes or inflammation can cause redness on the face that may appear to be rosacea. When the steroids are stopped, the redness usually resolves.

Signs and symptoms: Characterized by transient or persistent redness on the face, rosacea also may manifest as visible blood vessels, roughness, and pimple-like bumps on the face. As the disorder progresses, the skin gets even more inflamed and irregular in appearance. In extreme cases, rosacea may cause the "W. C. Fields nose," or rhinophyma.

Prevention and treatment: When rosacea is first diagnosed, it is important to understand which cleansers are best to use. It is important to avoid any skin care product that has a fragrance, as well as scrubs, abrasive materials, and other harsh exfoliants. I also recommend avoiding extreme temperatures for bathing and cleansing the face. Instead, use tepid water for washing and rinsing.

Other common triggers to watch out for include emotional stress, sun exposure, hot weather, cold weather, wind, humidity, heavy exercise, hot baths, alcohol, and spicy foods, among others. In one National Rosacea Society survey, researchers found that 81 percent of the patients surveyed said that the top trigger for rosacea flare-ups was sunlight. Sunscreen with a sun protection factor (SPF) of at least 15 must be used 365 days a year to prevent rosacea outbreaks. In addition, red wine has a natural pigment that tends to redden the skin tissue on the face and forehead in patients with rosacea. Avoidance of red wine is often recommended during rosacea flares.

Topical antibiotics and metronidazole, an antifungal, are frequently used as initial therapy for rosacea. Metronidazole has been shown to have anti-inflammatory and other healing properties, but it has limited success with rosacea. The topical treatment may be combined with a short course of oral antibiotics during the early stages of inflammatory lesions. Because demodex mites are thought to play a role in rosacea, the acaricides, chemical agents such as permethrin cream, are used in some cases. Lindane lotion, a common treatment for scabies and head and body lice, is also used for patients who do not respond to topical or oral antibiotics.

Oral antibiotics such as tetracycline, doxycycline, and erythromycin are often prescribed for patients with the more serious nodular rosacea and are indicated in patients with ocular symptoms. It usually takes up to six weeks for improvement to be shown with topical therapy, so oftentimes ointments are used in combination with oral therapy. The oral medication is then slowly withdrawn.

When to call the doctor: Check with your doctor upon the first signs of rosacea, when treatment is most effective. If you have lived with unmanaged rosacea for a period of time, it is important to have your skin medically evaluated and see if a stronger medication may be warranted.

Pregnancy Mask (Melasma)

What is it? Because of hormonal changes in a pregnant woman, the skin on her face will sometimes darken, forming a "masklike" effect. Called melasma, this condition commonly occurs on the forehead, chin, and upper lip, and is most prevalent in women with darker complexions. It usually appears during the second or third trimester of pregnancy. The pigmentation gradually fades after delivery, and will likely darken again with each subsequent pregnancy.

What causes it? While the exact cause of melasma is unknown, it is thought that pregnancy, oral contraceptives, cosmetics, genetics, sun exposure, and certain illnesses and medications can all contribute to the pigmentary change in the skin. Blotchy hyperpigmentation can also be caused by acne, eczema, contact dermatitis, and skin injuries, among other conditions.

Who's at risk? Melasma affects about 75 percent of pregnant women. Women who have melasma that is unrelated to pregnancy or oral contraceptive use may have hormone imbalances.

Signs and symptoms: Melasma causes splotchy areas of hyperpigmentation on the face. With melasma, tan or dark brown patches that are irregular in shape usually develop on the upper cheek, lips, and forehead.

Prevention and treatment: Use a broad-spectrum SPF sunblock to prevent malasma from worsening. Over-the-counter hydroquinone (page 51) preparations are often used to treat this condition, helping to fade the darkened pigmentation. Prescription-strength (4 percent) hydroquinone is a chemical that inhibits tyrosinase, an enzyme involved in the production of melanin. Azelaic acid (20 percent) is thought to decrease the activity of melanocytes, cells that produce melanin. Some women benefit from facial peels that use the stronger percentage of alpha hydroxy acids or chemical peels with glycolic acid.

When to call the doctor: If the hyperpigmentation is new or has worsened, talk with your doctor and get a medical diagnosis. Your doctor may wish to prescribe a stronger treatment or do tests to assess the cause, such as a hormone imbalance.

Moles (Nevi)

What is it? A nevus or mole is a benign tumor of melanocytes. The number of moles peaks in early adulthood and then decreases over a lifetime.

What causes it? Moles are the result of a harmless proliferation of pigment cells deep within the skin. Congenital nevi are moles you are born with (birthmarks).

Who's at risk? Almost everyone has moles. Between 5 and 10 percent of the white adult population of the United States (about 15 to 30 million people) have abnormal moles. These moles have the potential to progress into malignant melanoma, although the risk is relatively low — except in those individuals who have family members with malignant melanoma.

The size of moles is very important, because those larger than six millimeters in diameter have a greater chance of developing skin cancer. Those individuals who have many moles or atypical moles are at higher risk of melanoma, the most serious form of skin cancer. The risk factors for developing melanoma are both genetic and environmental, with sun exposure considered to be the major modifiable risk factor (one you can control). Other risk factors include:

- A new mole or change in an existing mole
- Family history of melanoma
- Personal history of basal cell or squamous cell cancer
- More than ten atypical nevi or a high number of normal nevi (more than fifty)
- Immunosuppression
- History of excessive sun exposure, inability to tan, and sun-induced freckles
- Blistering sunburns in the first two decades of life
- Caucasian
- Red or blond hair; green or blue eyes

Signs and symptoms: Moles can range in color from flesh tone to red pink to brown, tan, or, less often, black. They do not have a "stuck on" or wartlike appearance, and they are not scaly like other skin conditions. Melanomas usually have a blurring of borders, asymmetry, and a history of changing.

Prevention and treatment: Large congenital moles have an increased risk for the development of malignant melanoma. Melanoma is the sixth most common skin cancer in Americans and the most fatal malignancy among young adults. But melanoma is curable if detected and properly treated during the earliest phase of development. The best treatment for congenital moles is a surgical procedure. For those that are very large, cryosurgery or dermabrasion may help.

When to call the doctor: If you have a new mole or a change in an existing mole, call your doctor for an evaluation. Also, if you have more than ten atypical moles or more than fifty normal moles, see your doctor for a screening. With early detection, most cases of melanoma are curable.

Know the ABCDEs of Melanoma

Asymmetry
Border irregularities
Color variegation (i.e., different colors within the same region)
Diameter greater than 6 mm
Enlargement

Skin Concerns for the Thirties

During this decade, women may notice that their skin is drier and duller in appearance. This is because of the slowdown in new cells being produced. There is also an increase in tiny lines and wrinkles that can be subtle or obvious, depending on health and lifestyle habits. Some women notice sagging skin in the neck, chin, and jowl areas. At this stage in the life cycle, they may also have more cellulite, fat stores underneath the skin.

During the thirties, you may be at risk for certain skin conditions such as rosacea. Women in their thirties should avoid excess exposure to UV sun rays and other harsh environmental conditions (both hot and cold temperatures). Also, stay away from first- and secondhand smoke, as this can contribute to premature skin aging.

Fine Lines and Wrinkles

What is it? In normal skin aging, around age thirty, the production of collagen and elastin fibers is diminished and skin cell turnover begins to slow down, resulting in the appearance of fine lines and wrinkles and a sallow complexion.

What causes it? As discussed in chapter 2, you can blame your age, genetics, and gravity, but photoaging is the preeminent cause of early lines and wrinkles. In normal (intrinsic) aging, there is a loss of elastin fibers, which results in fine wrinkles. These shallow wrinkles disappear as the skin stretches. By age fifty, when the skin's elasticity declines dramatically, the powerful effect of gravity becomes more apparent and wrinkles are permanent, along with other signs such as elongation of the ears, extra folds of skin around the neck, and jowls along the jawline.

Who's at risk? Any woman who has a history of photodamage can have fine lines and wrinkles. This increases with age. Smoking, sleep positions, and facial expressions also increase the chance of wrinkles.

Signs and symptoms: With normal aging, the epidermis (outer skin layer) becomes thin, fragile, and inelastic. There is a gradual loss of blood vessels, fat, collagen, and elastin fibers. A reduction in the density of hair follicles, sweat ducts, and sebaceous (oil) glands results in a reduction of perspiration and sebum production.

With photoaging, the skin takes on a thickened, leathery look and is characterized by elastosis (coarsening and yellow discoloration). Wrinkles become deep and do not disappear with stretching, as they do with intrinsic aging. Not only does the sun cause early wrinkles, it also results in loss of elasticity in the walls of the tiny blood vessels that feed the skin, which can result in the formation of telangiectasia, or spider veins (page 194). With photoaging, there is irregular pigmentation, roughness and/or dryness, and often benign or malignant neoplasms (tumors).

Skin that has been protected from the sun's UV rays springs back quickly when touched or pinched, but sun-weakened skin does not. The more skin is exposed to sunlight, the greater the tendency toward premature wrinkles and a leathery complexion.

Prevention and treatment: The best way to prevent premature fine lines and wrinkles is to change your lifestyle habits, as discussed in steps 1 through 6. Although you cannot change the photodamage from the past, you can eat a diet rich in antioxidants, the compounds that attack free radicals in the body and destroy them. Exercise moderately and avoid the damaging effects of extreme hot or cold temperatures. Get healing sleep and prevent the ravages of

life's stressors from robbing you of sexy, ageless skin. Most important, start today to avoid the UV rays of the sun.

If you are going outdoors, avoid the sun's strongest hours,
10:00 a.m. to 3:00 p.m. When you go out in the sun, always wear a
sunscreen with an SPF of at least 15 and reapply it every two hours.
If you live in the South, spend time out of doors, have fair skin, or
have a history of skin cancer in your family, use sun products with
an SPF of at least 30 and apply it hourly or as often as it takes to prevent your skin from turning pink. Also, don't smoke, as this accelerates the normal aging process of the skin. Even after only ten years
of smoking, the skin changes and wrinkles are irreversible.

Treatments of the lines and wrinkles associated with photoaged
skin include topical vitamin A acid and alpha hydroxy acids. Other
treatments include products that contain natural moisturizing
ingredients such as Bio-Maple, urea, lactic acid, carboxylic acid,
sodium pyrollidone, and phospholipids.

When to call the doctor: If the photodamage is severe, talk to
your doctor about a chemical peel, dermabrasion, or laser treatment.

Under-eye Circles

While there are many causes of under-eye circles, the main ones are
blood vessels that show underneath the skin and skin that is hyper-
pigmented because of photodamage. Other causes include allergies,
genetics, fatty deposits, and aging.

To treat under-eye circles, use ingredients such as vitamin K,
silica, hesperetin, and vitamin C ester.

Skin Tags (Acrochordon)

What is it? Skin tags are an outgrowth of normal skin that can
occur almost anywhere for no reason at all. They appear frequently
on the eyelids, armpits, shoulders, neck, and groin of adults age
thirty-five and over.

What causes it? There is no exact cause, although we know that
skin tags have a genetic component and occur at sites of friction.

Who's at risk? Skin tags occur in about 25 percent of adults,
and their occurrence increases with age until about age fifty. Skin

tags also occur frequently during the second trimester of pregnancy and may regress postpartum. They appear to run in families and are common in individuals with Crohn's disease (an inflammatory bowel disease).

Signs and symptoms: Skin tags begin as tiny pieces of brown-colored skin attached to short stalks. They can become irritated if rubbed by clothing or jewelry and often turn red or black if the blood supply is cut off.

Prevention and treatment: The skin tag stalks can be removed by excising them with surgical scissors, cryosurgery with liquid nitrogen, or by electrocautery.

When to call the doctor: If the skin tag is irritated, bleeds, or tears, call your doctor for removal. Larger skin tags may need sutures after removal.

Décolleté Health

It's easy to neglect protecting the skin of the neck and chest. Yet even at a young age, these areas can appear aged and wrinkled, with mottled, uneven skin tone, skin laxity, and a roughened appearance.

Always protect this often uncovered area with sunscreen and moisturize with film-forming preparations that have ingredients such as petrolatum, ceramides, squalane, phospholipids, and vitamin E.

Skin Concerns for the Forties

You may notice drier skin during your early forties, along with more wrinkles around the eyes (crow's-feet) and mouth (lip lines). Try an alpha hydroxy acid (AHA) to slough off the dead skin cells. Follow with a multipurpose moisturizer containing petrolatum, squalane, urea, sodium lactate, hyaluronic acid, sodium PCA, or Bio-Maple.

Perimenopausal Skin

What is it? Perimenopause occurs in the two to eight years prior to menopause (during the early to late forties for most women). At this time, estrogen levels first start their decline, resulting in various physiological changes.

What causes it? This transition period prior to menopause is caused by a decline in estrogen. Symptoms occur as the woman's body adjusts to the reduced level of hormones.

Who's at risk? All women who have a natural transition into menopause will go through perimenopause, with its vague to intrusive signs and symptoms. Women who undergo a surgical hysterectomy and "medical menopause" do not go through this moderate transitory period.

Signs and symptoms: At this time, women may begin to notice that tiny lines become more pronounced and small creases become permanent wrinkles. This period is when women first notice the early signs of sagging skin, enlarged pores, and significant blotchiness, skin mottling, and extreme dryness. While it is not as common as other signs, many women in their forties suffer with adult acne.

Prevention and treatment: During perimenopause, women should begin regular anti-aging treatments, including daily use of eye cream, antioxidant day cream, mild skin cleansers, and weekly exfoliation to reveal clearer, brighter-looking skin.

When to call the doctor: If you notice dramatic skin changes during this period, talk with your doctor. Some women take low-dose birth control pills to help ease the symptoms during perimenopause, but most women recognize the signs and make lifestyle changes that help them cope.

Liver Spots (Solar Lentigo)

What is it? Liver spots, or age spots, are brown spots caused by chronic (long-term) sun exposure.

Who's at risk? Fair-skinned individuals who have spent a great deal of time in the sun are at higher risk for liver spots, as are those with an inherited tendency.

Signs and symptoms: Liver spots are sharply defined, round or oval, brown or black flat patches of skin most commonly seen on the backs of the hands or on the face. The spots may appear singly or clustered together. The hyperpigmentation is uniform within each spot and varies from light to dark brown. The spots can be as large as several inches or as small as a quarter of an inch. They are most noticeable on the hands, face, shoulders, and back (those areas that have had chronic sun exposure).

Prevention and treatment: Therapeutic treatment to fade liver spots includes bleaching creams, topical vitamin A acid, hydroquinone, and alpha hydroxy acids. Be sure to wear sunscreen at all times to keep the faded areas from darkening again.

When to call the doctor: Liver spots are not cancerous, but they can be accompanied by precancerous scaly red elevations of the skin called actinic keratoses. Actinic keratoses are premalignant lesions that develop only on sun-damaged skin, in contrast to basal cell carcinomas (BCC), which can occur on skin that has not been exposed to the sun.

Crow's-Feet

What is it? The term *crow's-feet* is usually associated with fine lines and wrinkles in the corners of and around the eyes.

What causes it? This common problem appears after years of squinting, sun exposure, lifestyle abuse, and cigarette smoking.

Who's at risk? All women are at risk, but particularly those who are over thirty, smoke cigarettes, and don't protect their eyes from UV radiation with sunglasses. Women who live in places where the sun's rays are intense (Florida, California, Texas, and Hawaii) are at highest risk for crow's-feet.

Signs and symptoms: Tiny, thin lines (wrinkles) that extend from the outer edge of the eye toward the side hairline. These lines are accentuated upon smiling or any time the cheek lifts the eye area upward.

Prevention and treatment: Daily use of sunscreen, proper moisturizing, wearing a wide-brimmed hat, and wearing appropriate sunglasses are all a must. Treatment of existing lines includes topical emollients and humectants such as petrolatum, glycerin, Bio-Maple, squalane, antioxidants, vitamin A, alpha hydroxy acid, and skin laser for more severe cases.

Eczema

What is it? Often called dermatitis, eczema is a group of skin conditions that affects all age groups. While there are treatments to calm the symptoms, currently there is no "cure" for this common skin problem.

What causes it? It is a recurring, long-term inflammation of the skin that is related to sensitivity to allergens in the environment that are relatively harmless to others. Atopic eczema, the most common form, is linked to asthma and hay fever. Allergic contact dermatitis is caused by the body's reaction to a substance in contact with the skin — for example, eczema due to contact with nickel in earrings. Irritant contact dermatitis is caused by frequent contact with everyday substances such as detergents and chemicals that are irritating to the skin. This is most commonly found on adult hands. Adult seborrheic eczema affects adults ages twenty to forty and is caused by a yeast growth. This type is usually seen on the scalp as mild dandruff but can also spread to the face, ears, and chest. Varicose eczema affects the lower legs of adults in middle and old age.

Who's at risk? Because eczema is often a hereditary condition, it is genetically linked and runs in families. Anyone can get eczema, from infants to elderly adults.

Signs and symptoms: A mild form of eczema is dry, hot, and itchy. In severe cases, the skin is broken, raw, and bleeding. While eczema looks unpleasant, it is not contagious. Untreated, it can result in a skin ulcer.

Prevention and treatment: Although there is no cure for eczema, there are many ways to minimize the discomfort. Treatments can be over-the-counter or prescription and include emollients, topical steroids, oral steroids, and topical immunomodulators. Topical steroids (cortisone) are used on most types of eczema to reduce inflammation when it flares and the skin becomes inflamed. These ointments and creams come in several strengths, depending on the age of patient, the severity of the condition, and the size of the area to be treated. If topical steroids are ineffective, oral steroids can be prescribed by a physician for more severe cases. Topical immunomodulators, substances that help to regulate the immune system, are used sometimes when eczema is particularly difficult to manage.

When to call the doctor: If the inflamed, irritated skin is new and you have not received a diagnosis, it is best to talk to your doctor. Also, if the eczema is difficult to manage through avoidance of the trigger or with over-the-counter moisturizers and creams, your doctor can best guide you in how to treat it.

Lip Lines

What is it? Lip lines or wrinkles are common among women over age thirty-five, and can be very frustrating, as they disrupt what would be a smooth upper lip line.

What causes it? Lip lines are the result of both chronological and environmental factors, including health problems, overexposure to the sun's rays, smoking, dry or overheated working and living conditions, and even the herpes virus.

Who's at risk? Most women over age thirty-five are at risk for lip lines. This risk increases with age, a history of photodamage, a dry environment, exposure to the sun, cigarette smoking, and excessive dieting.

Signs and symptoms: Lip lines are tiny vertical lines that extend from the top of the lip line upward. When lipstick is applied, the tiny lines become even more noticeable as the applied color bleeds upward toward the nose.

Prevention and treatment: The lips demand special consideration because they lack sebaceous glands and are prone to becoming chapped and fissured. Avoid the sun and cigarette smoking. Pursing the lips when smoking can leave permanent lip lines.

Treatment for lip lines includes the judicious use of topical emollients and sunblocks. To prevent lip lines from worsening, apply lip balm often, starting twenty minutes before sun exposure, and reapply several times throughout the day. Look for a lip-protecting therapy containing emollients such as petrolatum, oils (such as safflower), waxes (such as carnauba and paraffin), and sunblocks containing zinc, titanium oxide, oxybenzone, octinoxate, and benzophenone.

When to call the doctor: If a lip sore does not heal after several days or a lesion with a crusty edge develops, consult your doctor immediately.

Skin Concerns for the Fifties and Beyond

Menopausal Skin

What is it? Menopause is a normal life transition that usually occurs around age fifty-one. A woman's body undergoes a number of changes in metabolism, hormone production, and the length and frequency of menstrual periods, among other things. Twenty years ago, menopause (referred to at the time as "the change") was practically off-limits in conversation. Fortunately, attitudes toward this passage have changed.

What causes it? It is thought that the hormones estrogen and progesterone play a role in keeping skin healthy. Estrogen levels have a direct effect on the plenitude and thickness of collagen and elastin, the firming tissues that help support the structure of the skin. Therefore, decreasing levels of estrogen and progesterone induced by menopause can often contribute to the skin's poorer appearance. The onset of menopause may cause collagen levels to decrease by as much as 2 percent per year, contributing to slower wound healing and the appearance of more wrinkles.

Who's at risk? All women will go through menopause at some point in their lives. Women of any age who undergo a surgical hysterectomy with removal of the uterus and both ovaries will undergo a "medical menopause" at that time.

Signs and symptoms: During menopause, about 75 percent of women experience hot flashes (or flushes), a sudden and unexpected feeling of heat all over the body, generally starting around the head and neck, and they can affect a woman's skin, making it feel flushed, irritated, and rough. Sweating is a part of the hot flash. The flashes most often begin in the perimenopausal period, when relative estrogen deficiency first starts to occur along with cycle irregularity. Some women do not notice hot flashes until after menopause. Then there are women who have no signs of hot flashes at all.

Along with feeling flushed, many women begin to notice drier skin and changes in pigmentation during menopause. Decreased cutaneous collagen results in thinner skin with less elasticity, especially for women who have spent a great deal of time in the sun in younger years. Because of the decline in estrogen, menopausal women are also at higher risk of osteoporosis (bone loss), with fractures. Osteoporosis can result in sagging skin on the face.

Other skin changes at menopause include:

- A reduction in the ability of the skin to protect itself against UV radiation

- A decline in the enzymes necessary for collagen stabilization
- A reduction in the amount of sweat secretion and sebaceous gland output, contributing to the generalized dryness and roughness characteristic of aging skin
- A decrease in vitamin D production (necessary for strong bones and preventing fractures)
- A decrease in blood vessels and blood circulation in the skin
- A change in the rate of hair growth; hair often thins in some areas but may also grow thicker in other areas
- A change in hair color

Prevention and treatment: Even though changes associated with skin aging cannot be reversed, there are numerous avenues of treatment open to slow down the aging process and reverse some of the tissue damage. The skin should also be protected from the damaging effects of the environment, particularly solar UV radiation. Because incremental damage occurs with each exposure to UV light, it's increasingly necessary to avoid the sun, wear protective clothing, and use sunscreen. Damage can occur even when there is no evidence of sunburn on the skin.

As you read product labels, be sure to look for ingredients that combat uneven skin tone and penetrate into the stratum corneum (the outer layer of the skin) to form a film on the skin and to lock in moisture. Some of these ingredients include powerful, natural moisturizing factor compounds such as hyaluronic acid, urea, Bio-Maple, lactic acid, sodium hyaluronate, sodium lactate, cholesterol, phytoesterols, salicylic acid, sphingolipids and phospholipids, alpha hydroxy acids (AHAs) and beta hydroxy acids (BHAs), glycerin, antioxidants, and sunscreens.

When to call the doctor: If you notice any skin changes that are new or different, see your doctor. At this stage in the life cycle, get a thorough skin evaluation annually to avoid more serious types of skin cancer or diseases.

Spider Veins (Telangiectasia)

Spider veins (telangiectasia) are normal veins that have dilated under the influence of venous pressure. These small, superficial veins enlarge and appear as a "sunburst" pattern of reddish and purplish veins. Spider veins are more common in women than in men and usually start in childhood. Although the veins rarely bleed, they do represent a cosmetic problem. They are treated by electrodesiccation or laser treatment. They may also be disguised with makeup.

Skin Cancer (Carcinomas)

What is it? The most common form of skin cancer is basal cell carcinoma — a cancer that develops in the basal layer of the skin, deeper than the surface layer. It is associated with aging and years of chronic sun exposure. Basal cell carcinoma seldom spreads to other parts of the body, but it can be disfiguring if not treated early. Some symptoms are translucent pearly bumps on sun-exposed skin. They often crust, ulcerate, and bleed, and are sometimes confused with ordinary pimples. Although basal cell carcinoma has little chance of spreading (metastasizing) via blood and lymph systems, it can cause extensive skin destruction and should not be ignored.

Squamous cell carcinoma is the second most common form of skin cancer. Skin symptoms are elevated opaque bumps that may appear mushroom- or wartlike and take on a pink coloration. The lesions may ulcerate and become infected. They are often found on the lips, face, hands, and rims of the ears. Squamous cell carcinoma is capable of spreading to other organs and should be immediately referred to a dermatologist as soon as symptoms are detected.

The least common but the most serious skin cancer is malignant melanoma, which is capable of metastasizing via lymph and blood systems. The most common sites for melanoma are the neck, upper head, trunk, and lower extremities. Melanoma lesions look like moles that are flat with indistinct or irregular borders and have varying colors such as brown, blue, white, black, and red. The incidence and diagnosis of malignant melanoma have increased dramatically, and no one is immune, including individuals with dark skin color.

What causes it? The main cause of skin cancer is ultraviolet (UV) radiation from the sun. UV rays damage DNA. If the genetic damage is severe, normal skin cells begin to grow in an abnormal, disorderly way, like other types of cancer cells. Sometimes skin cancer is genetically linked and is caused by abnormal genes that are inherited.

Who's at risk? Anyone of any race can get skin cancer, including the very serious melanoma. Individuals are at highest risk of skin cancer if they have blond or red hair, blue or green eyes, sunburn easily, and/or have a family history of skin cancer.

Signs and symptoms: Early warnings of skin cancer include the appearance of new growth or the change in size, color, or shape of a skin lesion. You may also notice the development of crust, scabs, or bleeding within a supposed mole, a supposed freckle, a wart, or a liver spot, with accompanying pain and itching in or around these lesions.

Prevention and treatment: Prevention begins with avoiding exposure to the sun's ultraviolet rays. Sunscreen, sunglasses, wide-brimmed hats, and avoidance of the sun's strongest rays (between 10:00 a.m. and 3:00 p.m.) are the best ways to keep your skin cancer free.

When to call the doctor: If you notice any change in a mole, freckle, wart, or liver spot, call your doctor for an evaluation. If you have many moles or a family history of skin cancer, talk to a dermatologist about "mole mapping," a procedure that involves digital imaging, archiving, and diagnosis of moles and other suspicious lesions. This is especially important for those of European descent and those with a family or personal history of skin cancer, excessive exposure to the sun (especially during childhood), and many large or unusual moles. Regular follow-up examinations and scans allow the doctor to compare the earlier scans and make a diagnosis at an early stage, when treatment is most effective.

Diabetes and Skin Problems

People with diabetes experience a wide array of skin problems. Some are triggered by the medications necessary to treat the illness, and others include infections that can be life threatening. Problems associated with this disease include thickening of the skin, yellowing of the skin, and the appearance of small round colored spots on the lower legs. Talk to a doctor to determine the severity of your skin symptoms if you have diabetes.

Understanding Postmenopausal Skin

Postmenopause (sixties and beyond), the amount of sebum (oil) produced by the skin declines up to 50 percent. The result is dry skin, and many women at this life stage experience skin splits and cracks. There are also more sun spots, spider veins, and facial sagging. Skin blotchiness and spider veins on the neck and chest (called poikiloderma) are a direct result of sun damage. Postmenopausal women should follow the same skin care recommendations as women with menopausal skin (pages 192–193).

Beyond Botox Recommendations for Radiate

1. Taking care of common and more serious skin problems when they first appear can keep skin healthy and ageless.

2. Understanding the causes, the risk factors, the signs and symptoms, and the various ways to prevent and treat skin problems can prevent more serious complications.

3. Each stage in the life cycle brings with it new skin changes and concerns. Knowing what changes to look out for enables you to treat these problems early on, avoiding more costly and invasive treatments.

4. If a skin problem is new, see your doctor for a proper diagnosis and medical treatment, if needed.

Conclusion

Over the past few years, there have been important advances and new information relating to the architecture and biochemistry of the skin. Improved vehicles, humectants, have led to new and exciting treatment opportunities, which are constantly evolving. No longer is it acceptable to offer a pleasant-smelling topical preparation that feels good on the skin and accomplishes very little.

The reality is that we are judged by our complexion and the way we look. Another reality is that nowadays, most of us live longer and are healthier to a more advanced age. Ergo, beware the craziness surrounding elective, invasive medical procedures that promise a mythical fountain of youth but deliver little. Fortunately, there are other alternatives out there. For the first time, we can offer multi-functional preparations that yield excellent benefits treating environmentally compromised skin without the drawbacks of expensive, quick-fix injections.

In this volume, I've tried to convey the very practical notions of a healthy, intelligent lifestyle together with a realistic, responsible program that eliminates the need for buying into the marketing boom around suspect procedures. Botox certainly isn't for everybody. There exist today other, less onerous options geared to a better-informed public. Women *do* have better choices for a more intelligent approach. I urge you to follow the B. Kamins seven-step program; it will help both you and your skin feel young again!

Ben Kaminsky

Acknowledgments

We want to thank Debra Fulghum Bruce, PhD, who when we first approached her with the concept believed in us and the book. Deb, you are a true professional. You helped mold our thoughts and translate them into a focused book. Your hard work and dedication and experience were invaluable. Your work ethic is impeccable, and you're truly a model for us to emulate.

We also want to thank Denise Marcil, whose professional help and good sense guided us to realize this project.

Our thanks to Karen Murgolo, vice president and associate publisher of Springboard Press, and Michelle Howry, senior editor, Springboard Press, who immediately understood our vision and guided us with their years of experience. You both have a keen eye and were a pleasure to work with. Also to Jill Cohen, publisher of Springboard Press, and Maureen Egen, publisher of Hachette Book Group USA, for your support in publishing the book. From the moment we met you both, we knew that we were involved with nice, caring people.

There are so many other people who deserve thanks, but unfortunately we do not have the space to specifically acknowledge everybody here. Please know that our appreciation for your efforts is heartfelt and sincere.

Ben and Howard Kaminsky

Ben's acknowledgments

I owe a huge debt to my wife, Mildred, for being patient and kind to me during the many hours I spent trying to write a responsible, slim book about my passion to better understand healthy skin care. Even though Mildred benefited mightily from the work in the lab, she nonetheless was my greatest critic and muse. What a great lady!

This whole project would not have occurred without the energy and persistence of my older son, Howard. His passion, perseverance, and work ethic are gigantic. He deserves all the kudos and success he has achieved. My daughter, Gila, and son David did not hesitate to set me straight about "too much use of scientific jargon that is heavy and eggheaded."

I also want to thank Herbert Nemteanu of our quality control/ regulatory department, who spent hours with me sorting, organizing, and editing concepts and text.

Ben Kaminsky

Howard's acknowledgments

I would like to thank my beloved wife, Laurie, who's always helped me make my dreams come true and supported me even through the long working hours. To my daughter, Isabelle, who inspires me every day and keeps my skin care passion alive. To my other child, whom Laurie is carrying, I can't wait to meet you.

A special thanks to Candace Solomon, MS, for insight into feng shui techniques to enhance rest and relaxation.

To our B. Kamins staff members Annabelle Eggleton, Claire Labrom, and Joe Fotheringham, thank you for your help. And, my thanks to the entire team at B. Kamins, Chemist, for being the most responsible and professional skin care group in the industry.

Most important, I want to thank my father, whose convictions and professional ethics and integrity have been role models from day one. Dad, your sense of priorities and values, even though it is a daunting task, is one I wish to emulate and pass on. I remember you spending hours in the lab after I complained about a sunburn, formulating a sunscreen for me. Dad, I know in my heart you agreed to start B. Kamins not as a business opportunity but as a way to give me a business and for us to work together. I thank you and love you.

Howard Kaminsky

Appendix I:

Resources

Readers can find more information on skin care and spas at the following associations' Web sites and in the following publications.

Associations

- American Massage Therapy Association (http://www.amta massage.org/): To find a licensed massage therapist and learn more on how massage therapy may help your situation.
- The Day Spa Association (http://www.dayspaassociation.com/): To find a day spa in your area and read articles about day spas.
- International Spa Association (http://www.experienceispa.com/ ISPA/): To search for a spa, to find a spa travel agent, and to read articles about the various types of spas.
- National Certification Board for Therapeutic Massage and Bodywork (http://www.ncbtmb.com): To find certified therapeutic massage and bodywork practitioners in your area.
- The Spa Association (http://www.thespaassociation.com/): To find articles and news events involving spas around the world and also to locate a spa.

Publications

- *American Spa* (http://www.americanspamag.com/american spa/): To read about the spa industry, including information on new and renovated spas around the United States and innovative products used at spas.

- *DAYSPA* (http://www.dayspamagazine.com/): To read articles on spa therapies and the spa industry.
- *Massage* (http://www.massagemag.com/): To read articles on the latest innovations in bodywork and massage therapies.

Or visit our Web site at www.beyondbotox.com.

Appendix II:

B. Kamins Products for Sexy, Ageless Skin

Product	Indications	Key Benefits	Key Ingredients
		Cleanse and Tone	
Vegetable Skin Cleanser	A vegetable-based cleanser and makeup remover for all skin types, including acne, acne-rosacea, eczema, and sensitive skin	Effectively dissolves and removes impurities from the face and the delicate eye area without overdrying and irritating skin	Lauryl glucoside, long chain sulfonated tensio-active agents, hydrolyzed soy protein, Bio-Maple compound (physiological humectant/moisturizer), almond glycerides, glycerin
Botanical Face Cleanser	A nonirritating emulsion cleanser ideal for removing dirt and oil from normal/combination skin	Cleans and rids the skin of excess sebum to reduce breakouts	Bio-Maple compound (physiological humectant/moisturizer), quillaja saponaria root extract, lecithin (phospholipids)
Vitamin Face Cleanser	A hydrating and polishing lotion specially formulated for drier skin types	Delicately exfoliates skin's surface while leaving it supple and hydrated. Provides antioxidant vitamin protection.	Olive fruit oil, sesame seed oil, glycerin, walnut shell powder, tocopheryl acetate (vitamin E), retinyl palmitate (vitamin A), soya sterols

Product	Indications	Key Benefits	Key Ingredients
Cleanse and Tone *(continued)*			
Hydrogen-Ion Moisturizing Toner Available for dry, normal/ combination, or oily skin	To hydrate and reionize skin to its normal pH balance	Gently exfoliates and conditions with plant extracts and moisturizers	Bio-Maple compound (physiological humectant/ moisturizer), glycolic acid, lactic acid, cucumber fruit extract, vitamin E
Bamboo & Rice Facial Polisher	A gentle, polishing, textured cleanser for all skin types	Helps clarify and refine sallow, thickened, sun-damaged, mottled, or acneic complexions	Lauryl glucoside, Bio-Maple compound (physiological humectant/moistur-izer), rice bran wax, bamboo stem powder, long chain tensio-active agents
Repair			
Cellular Renewal Serum	All skin types; for sun- and environmentally damaged, wrinkled, blotchy skin	Provides gentle exfoliation; helps restore clarity, radiance, and suppleness	Alpha hydroxy fruit acids, Bio-Maple compound (physiological humectant/moistur-izer), glycosamino-glycans (ceramides)
Revitalizing Booster Concentrate	For skin traumatized by laser, radiation, chemical peels, microdermabra-sion, and rosacea conditions	Allergy tested for the most sensitive skin. Soothes and calms irritated, reddened skin without clogging pores. Ideal for use after waxing and electrolysis treatments.	Anti-inflammatory bisabolol, moisturizing Bio-Maple compound (physiological humectant/ moisturizer), antioxidants, vitamins A and E, emollient squalane skin protection
Glycolic-6 / Glycolic-8 / Glycolic-10	Topical moisturizing exfoliants for face, neck, and décolleté	Helps increase the rate of cell renewal, revealing smoother, healthier-looking skin	Alpha hydroxy fruit acids, Bio-Maple compound (physiological humectant/ moisturizer)

Product	Indications	Key Benefits	Key Ingredients

Repair *(continued)*

Product	Indications	Key Benefits	Key Ingredients
Menopause Skin Cream (Nutrient Replacement Cream)	Perimenopausal and menopausal hormone-deprived skin symptoms, including excessive dryness, skin flushing and sweating, uneven tone, thinning of the skin resulting from diminished collagen and elastin synthesis	Antioxidant protection (anti-wrinkle), cooling action to control flushing, soothing effect to combat irritation due to excess sweating, powerful moisturizing ingredients to plump thinning skin, emollients to soften and help restore a normal stratum corneum	Episphere-Blue (polysaccharide encapsulated tocopherol and silica compound, anti-aging wrinkle protection and light-scattering reflection for dark circles, body heat extended-release delivery system), menthyl lactate, Bio-Maple compound (physiological humectant/moisturizer), Profusion Ceramide Complex (plumping and firming action), salicylic acid, horse chestnut extract, squalane
Skin-Lightening Treatment	For hyper-pigmented discolorations (brown patches), including sun spots and age spots	Helps to gradually fade brown spots resulting from both chronological and environmental skin damage	Hydroquinone, kojic acid, salicylic acid, stabilized vitamin C (magnesium ascorbyl phosphate), Bio-Maple compound (physiological humectant/ moisturizer)

Repair: *Anti-Aging*

Product	Indications	Key Benefits	Key Ingredients
Therapeutic Eye Cream	For dark circles around the eyes and skin bruising resulting from cosmetic skin procedures	Contains antioxidants' catalysts and tissue repair anti-aging compounds. Helps strengthen fragile capillaries, which may appear as dark patches in the eye area. Helps shorten	Copper and zinc oligopeptides, sodium hyaluronate, Bio-Maple compound (physiological humectant/moistur-izer), squalane, glycosaminoglycans, vitamins A, E, and K,

Product	Indications	Key Benefits	Key Ingredients
		Repair: Anti-Aging *(continued)*	
Therapeutic Eye Cream *(continued)*		the healing time for bruising caused by injections and other cosmetic surgical procedures.	hesperetin laurate, allantoin
Therapeutic Anti-Aging Wrinkle-Lift	An injection-free home treatment that targets wrinkles and expression lines	Creates an instant tightening, "lifting" sensation and helps firm and plump the skin, making wrinkles appear to lift and soften	Hydrolyzed soy protein, morus alba (mulberry) leaf extract, Bio-Maple compound (physiological humectant/ moisturizer), sodium PCA, glycerin, anti-aging zinc oligopeptides
Therapeutic Anti-Aging Moisturizer	For chronological and environmental skin-aging symptoms, particularly useful for treating photoaged, dry, wrinkled skin. Indicated to refine and lift fatigued, sallow complexions.	Multipurpose anti-aging cosmeceutical moisturizer that combines the most innovative anti-aging technologies with our exclusive Bio-Maple moisturizing compound. This treatment preparation is also recommended for long-term use both before and after cosmetic surgical procedures.	Amino oligopeptides (biological compounds/ wrinkle reducers), thioctic acid, grape seed oil, vitamins A and E (powerful anti-aging antioxidants), phosphatidylcholine (antioxidant), niacinamide (to increase microcirculation), bisabolol (anti-inflammatory/ antioxidant), urea, sodium lactate (natural moisturizing factors)

Product	Indications	Key Benefits	Key Ingredients

Repair: *Special Skin Needs: Rosacea*

Product	Indications	Key Benefits	Key Ingredients
Booster Blue Rosacea Cleanser	For all skin types, particularly formulated for rosacea and reddened/couperose skin conditions	Formulated with gentle, nonirritating tensio-active agents together with anti-inflammatory ingredients; fragrance free	Lauryl polyglucose (cleanser derived from vegetable corn source), cocoamphodiacetate (mild foaming cleanser derived from coconut oil), bisabolol (anti-inflammatory, anti-irritant, antifungal), Bio-Maple compound (physiological humectant/moisturizer)
Booster Blue Rosacea Treatment	For all skin types, particularly formulated for rosacea and reddened/couperose skin conditions	An emollient, anti-inflammatory rosacea treatment that helps to calm and soothe inflammation and dryness as well as cosmetically neutralize and reduce skin redness and blotchiness	Bisabolol (anti-inflammatory, anti-irritant, antifungal), squalane (lipid emollient moisturizer), vitamins A and E (antioxidant, anti-aging), Bio-Maple compound (physiological humectant/moisturizer)
Rosacea Moisturizer SPF 15	A gentle cosmetic emollient preparation that helps moisturize dry skin conditions associated with rosacea and related couperose (reddened) complexions	Helps moisturize and relieve inflammation and protects skin from UVA and UVB sun rays. May be used before and after makeup application.	UVA and UVB sunscreens (avobenzone, octinoxate, oxybenzone), Bio-Maple compound (physiological humectant/moisturizer), apricot kernel oil and soya sterols (to help moisturize, soften, and soothe irritated skin), vitamins A and E (for anti-wrinkle benefits)

Product	Indications	Key Benefits	Key Ingredients

Repair: *Special Skin Needs: Rosacea* (continued)

Product	Indications	Key Benefits	Key Ingredients
Booster Blue Rosacea Masque	For all skin types, particularly formulated for rosacea and reddened/couperose skin conditions	Helps to calm and soothe as well as cosmetically neutralize redness. Helps to gently desquamate hyperkeratotic (thickened) skin to provide a more uniform, brighter, and firmer complexion.	Bisabolol (anti-inflammatory, anti-irritant, antifungal), esculin (horse chestnut) (anti-inflammatory astringent), niacinamide (increases microcirculation, improves barrier function), Bio-Maple compound (physiological humectant/ moisturizer)

Repair: *Special Skin Needs: Acne*

Product	Indications	Key Benefits	Key Ingredients
Hydrating Acne Wash	For oily, combination, and normal skin types. To treat mild to moderate acne breakouts.	Helps to reduce blemishes; used to exfoliate dead skin cells and to emulsify excess skin oil to control breakouts	Salicylic acid (antibacterial, exfoliant, beta hydroxy acid), glycolic and lactic acid (exfoliants and moisturizers, alpha hydroxy acids), Bio-Maple compound (physiological humectant/moisturizer), allantoin (anti-irritant skin protectant), panthenol (humectant moisturizer)
Medicated Acne Gel Available in 5% and 10% strengths	For inflammatory and noninflammatory lesions, including blackheads, whiteheads, pustules (sores),	Helps to gently clear spots and blemishes, and to prevent the development of comedons/white-heads/blackheads.	Benzoyl peroxide (antibacterial topical medication), Bio-Maple compound (physiological humectant/ moisturizer), PEG

Product	Indications	Key Benefits	Key Ingredients

Repair: *Special Skin Needs: Acne (continued)*

Product	Indications	Key Benefits	Key Ingredients
Medicated Acne Gel *(continued)*	and papules (bumps). Available in 5% and 10% strengths to treat mild to moderate or severe acne breakouts.	Almost invisible upon application; oil-free, nondrying Bio-Maple hydrating formula.	dimethicone sulfosuccinate (oil-free emollient), carbomer (colorless water-dispersible gel base)
Matte Moisturizer SPF 15	A light, comforting daytime moisturizer, ideal for hydrating acne-prone skin	An oil-free, fragrance-free milky lotion that provides skin with a blend of moisturizers, vitamins, and antioxidants to condition and hydrate without clogging pores and causing breakouts. Provides sun protection.	UVA and UVB sunscreen protection (avobenzone, octinoxate, octisalate), Bio-Maple compound (physiological humectant/moisturizer), hydrolyzed elastin and marine proteins (for skin firming), vitamins A and E (for anti-wrinkle benefits)

Repair: *Special Skin Needs: Eczema*

Product	Indications	Key Benefits	Key Ingredients
Antipruritic Cream	To treat irritation and itching due to eczema, dermatitis, and allergies to jewelry, cosmetics, soaps, or detergents	Temporary relief of minor skin irritations, itching, and redness of the skin	Zinc oxide, squalane, glycerin, petrolatum, Bio-Maple compound (physiological humectant/moisturizer), menthyl lactate, allantoin, bisabolol, lecithin

Repair: *Special Skin Needs: Extradry Skin*

Product	Indications	Key Benefits	Key Ingredients
Maple Treatment Creamy Cleanser	To cleanse, moisturize, and soothe very dry to normal skin	Cleanses skin without stripping or overdrying. Softens and conditions with emollient oils to help improve skin's	Olive and sesame oils (emollients), Bio-Maple compound (physiological humectant/moisturizer), vitamins A and

Product	Indications	Key Benefits	Key Ingredients

Repair: *Special Skin Needs: Extradry Skin* (continued)

Product	Indications	Key Benefits	Key Ingredients
Maple Treatment Creamy Cleanser *(continued)*		natural elasticity and resiliency. Helps skin maintain its natural moisture barrier.	E (for anti-wrinkle benefits), octyl dodecanol (emulsifier/tensio-active agent)
Maple Treatment Day Cream SPF 15	For dry skin types, including parched skin conditions due to both chronological and environmental skin aging	Formulated to replenish skin's natural moisture level; serves as a healthy protective shield without leaving a heavy or greasy feel. SPF 15, UVA and UVB sunscreens provide protection against photoaging skin deterioration.	Broad-spectrum UVA and UVB sunscreens, Bio-Maple compound (physiological humectant/moistur-izer), soy sterols (to soothe and moisturize), soluble collagen (to increase skin plumpness), vitamins A and E (for anti-wrinkle benefits)
Maple Treatment Night Cream	To treat and rehydrate extremely dry skin. To supplement the skin's natural oils when they are depleted as a result of the aging process, sun damage, or illness.	A superemollient hydrating dermatological skin cream that combines anti-aging properties to treat the driest of complexions. Helps to eliminate flakiness and minimizes dry patches to provide a smooth, even complexion. Helps to restore the skin's natural protection barrier.	NMF (natural moisturizing factors) ingredients, including urea, sodium PCA, sodium lactate, and niacinamide (to increase microcircu-lation); castor seed oil and squalane (natural emollients and lubricating agents); Bio-Maple compound (physiological humectant/moistur-izer); and petrolatum (for skin occlusion and lubrication)

Product	Indications	Key Benefits	Key Ingredients
Moisturize			
Eye Cream	Fine lines, wrinkles, and dry skin tissue around the eye area	Helps reduce the appearance of fine lines, wrinkles, and dark circles while providing powerful antioxidant, anti-aging protection	Episphere-Blue (polysaccharide encapsulated tocopherol and silica compound, anti-aging wrinkle protection and light-scattering reflection for dark circles, body heat extended-release delivery system), Bio-Maple compound (physiological humectant/ moisturizer)
Day Lotion SPF 15	For oily to normal skin types, including acne-prone skin	An oil-free silky lotion that diffuses a blend of moisturizers, vitamins, and antioxidants into the inner layer of the epidermis to enhance day-long comfort and hydration without clogging pores and causing breakouts. Provides sun protection.	UVA and UVB sunscreen protection, Bio-Maple compound (physiological humectant/moistur-izer), marine protein and hydrolyzed elastin (for skin firming), vitamins A and E (for anti-wrinkle benefits)
Day Cream SPF 15	For normal to dry skin types. A perfect base for makeup application; for photoprotection, may be reapplied over makeup without smudging or distortion.	Helps restore skin's natural moisture level; serves as a protective shield against environmental assaults. Contains UVA and UVB sun protection factors. May be used before and after makeup application.	Broad-spectrum UVA and UVB sunscreens, Bio-Maple compound (physiological humectant/moistur-izer), apricot kernel oil and soy sterol (to help moisturize, soften, and soothe irritated skin), vitamins A and E (for anti-wrinkle benefits)

Product	Indications	Key Benefits	Key Ingredients

Moisturize *(continued)*

Product	Indications	Key Benefits	Key Ingredients
Night Cream	Perfect for normal to dry skin types. Helps restore and protect skin's moisture balance and supply essential nutrients, repair and rejuvenate skin's appearance.	A reparative treatment and antioxidant-rich formula that helps to diminish fine lines and wrinkles. Nongreasy, ultrahydrating formula.	Episphere-Blue (polysaccharide encapsulated tocopherol and silica compound, anti-aging wrinkle protection, body heat extended-release delivery system), Bio-Maple compound (physiological humectant/moisturizer), sodium hyaluronate and urea (powerful humectant moisturizers), apricot kernel oil and wheat germ oil, phoshatidylcholine and vitamin A (antioxidants)
Lip Balm SPF 20	For the prevention and treatment of cracked lips, lip lines, and sores. For smoothing lips before lipstick application (reduces the feathering effect).	An award-winning treatment balm that helps soothe dry lip conditions; helps prevent the formation of aging lip lines and the breakout of lip sores; contains UVA/UVB sunscreens. Protects lips from sun, wind, and extreme temperatures.	Wide-spectrum UVA/UVB protection with both physical and light-absorbing sunblocks, squalane, carnauba wax, caprilic/capric triglyceride (emollient softening and protecting agents), cyclopen-tasiloxane and dimethicone crosspolymer (silicone skin protection), vitamin A, and Bio-Maple compound (physiological humectant/ moisturizer)

Product	Indications	Key Benefits	Key Ingredients

Mask

Product	Indications	Key Benefits	Key Ingredients
Diatoma-mus Earth Masque Available for dry-to-normal or oily skin	Two hydrating botanical mask formulations available for dry-to-normal or oily skin types, formulated to remove the buildup of dead skin cells	Gentle exfoliating facial treatments created to hydrate, firm, nourish, and clarify while calming and soothing skin. Leaves skin smooth and luminous in appearance.	Diatomaceous earth (bentonite), Bio-Maple compound (physiological humectant/moisturizer), menthyl lactate (cooling agent), tocopherol nicotinate (stimulates microcirculation)
Therapeutic Brightening Masque	To fight the aging effects of skin glycation, such as mottled, yellowish, and wrinkled skin	Helps reduce the appearance of fine lines and improves skin tone, elasticity, and texture. Leaves skin smoother and brighter looking.	Bentonite, glycerin, glycolic acid, kaolin, safflower seed oil, squalane, Bio-Maple compound (physiological humectant/ moisturizer), anti-aging acetyl hexapeptide-3, kojic dipalmitate, soya sterols, vitamin E, magnesium ascorbyl phosphate, hydrolyzed elastin, marine protein

Protect from Sun

Product	Indications	Key Benefits	Key Ingredients
Sunbar Sunscreen SPF 30	For all skin types. To help reduce the signs of premature aging due to repeated and extended exposure to the sun over the years.	Wide-spectrum UVA and UVB protection with both physical and light-absorbing sunblocks. Ideal for rosacea or sensitive skin types and for fair-skinned individuals and patients who are taking photosensi-tizing medications. May be reapplied over makeup and should be used several times daily. Fragrance free.	Octinoxate and oxybenzone (benzophenone-3) (UVB sunscreens), avobenzone (UVA sunscreen), titanium dioxide (physical UVA and UVB sunscreen), polysiloxane (waterproofing ingredient), Bio-Maple compound (physiological humectant/ moisturizer)

Product	Indications	Key Benefits	Key Ingredients
	Protect from Sun (continued)		
Sunbar UVshield SPF 48	A high-protection sunblock formulated for fair or sun-sensitive skin types. Regular use helps reduce the signs of premature aging due to repeated and extended exposure to the sun.	Wide-spectrum UVA and UVB protection with both physical and light-absorbing sunblocks. Ideal for rosacea or sensitive skin types and for fair-skinned individuals and patients who are taking photosensitizing medications. May be reapplied over makeup and should be used several times daily. Fragrance and color free	Ensulizone, homosalate, octinoxate, octocrylene, zinc oxide, polysiloxane (waterproofing ingredient), dimethiconol, glycerin, lactic acid, Bio-Maple compound (physiological humectant/ moisturizer), vitamin E
	Body Care		
Body Lotion (Menopause)	Specially formulated for mature skin, including perimenopausal, menopausal, and postmenopause hormone-deprived skin types	Nongreasy formula that is ultramoisturizing and rehydrating. Formulated with soothing anti-itch cooling ingredients to help relieve excessive dryness, skin flushing, and sweating.	Oat protein (soothing and anti-itch), menthyl lactate (cooling agent), Profusion Ceramide Complex (sphingolipids and phospholipids), squalane and wheat germ oil (emollients), bisabolol (anti-inflammatory, anti-irritant, antifungal), Bio-Maple compound (physiological humectant/ moisturizer)

Product	Indications	Key Benefits	Key Ingredients
Body Care *(continued)*			
Elbow, Knee and Foot Treatment Kit Two-step kit: smoothing and polishing scrub and cellular exfoliating cream	For skin surface roughness and uneven skin coloration	Smoothes and polishes roughened, mottled skin and improves skin texture	Apricot seed powder, pumice, glycerin, PEG, Bio-Maple compound (physiological humectant/moisturizer), cocoglycerides, glycolic acid, morus nigra (mulberry) leaf extract, menthyl lactate
Flower Water Treatment Spray	An aromatic bouquet of flower scents for face and body	Rebalances and hydrates skin with pure glacier water and natural Bio-Maple compound	Glacier water, Bio-Maple compound (physiological humectant/moisturizer), citric acid, floral fragrance
Maple Sugar Body Scrub	A pampering body treatment for normal-to-dry dehydrated skin types	A luxurious emollient, senses-stimulating body treatment. Helps to exfoliate, brighten, and smooth dry, rough skin. Lubricates, softens, and moisturizes.	Bio-Maple sugar (exfoliant and moisturizing ingredient), sweet almond oil, sunflower oil, safflower oil (softening, moisturizing, vitamin-rich oils), vitamin E (antioxidant)
Maple Body Lotion	For all skin types. To replenish, protect, and soften skin all over the body.	A warmly scented therapeutic body lotion that absorbs quickly and pampers the body with rich shea butter, honey, vegetable oils, and extracts	Hyaluronic acid (potent humectant/moisturizer), shea butter (natural lipid and emollient), urea (moisturizer and anti-itch agent), jojoba oil and soy sterols (lubricants and moisturizers), honey, and Bio-Maple compound (physiological humectant/moisturizer)

Product	Indications	Key Benefits	Key Ingredients

Body Care *(continued)*

Product	Indications	Key Benefits	Key Ingredients
Maple Treatment Hand Cream SPF 20	For all skin types. Particularly recommended for very dry nail cuticles, hands, arms, and elbows.	A soothing, unscented moisturizing treatment cream that combats rough, dry skin and protects from damaging environmental factors such as sun, harsh climates, and drying detergents/cleansers. Absorbs rapidly. Helps prevent the formation of brown spots on the back of hands.	Octinoxate and octisalate (UVB sunscreens), avobenzone (UVA sunscreen), Bio-Maple compound (physiological humectant/moisturizer), urea (moisturizer and anti-itch agent), sodium lactate, honey extract, vitamins A and E (antioxidant, anti-aging)

Appendix III:

B. Kamins Cleansing and Moisturizing Guide

Skin Type	Best Product	Frequency	Follow Moisturizer
Normal	Vegetable Cleanser	AM	Day Cream SPF 15
		PM	Anti-Aging Therapeutic Moisturizer
Dry	Maple Treatment Creamy Cleanser	AM	Maple Treatment Day Cream SPF 15
		PM	Maple Treatment Night Cream
Oily	Botanical Cleanser	AM/PM	Day Lotion SPF 15
Pregnancy	Depends on skin type	AM/PM	Depends on skin type
Menopausal	Maple Treatment Creamy Cleanser	AM	Menopause Skin Cream
		PM	Anit-Aging Therapeutic Moisturizer
Acne	Hydrating Acne Wash	AM/PM	Matte Moisturizer SPF 15
Rosacea	Booster Blue Cleanser	AM/PM	Rosacea Moisturizer SPF 15

References and Supporting Research

The scientific studies and findings referenced in *Beyond Botox* are listed below by chapter.

Chapter 1

Habif TP. *Clinical Dermatology: A color guide to diagnosis and therapy.* New York: Mosby, 1996, v.

Botox may cause new wrinkles. BBC News World Edition, Feb 18, 2003.

Florida cites dangerous Botox clone in paralysis cases. *ScoutNews*, LLC, 2005.

Lin JY. α-Lipoic acid is ineffective as a topical anti-oxidant. *J Invest Dermatol* 2004; 123(5): 996–8.

American Heart Association recommendations from scientific sessions, 2004, http://www.americanheart.org/presenter.jhtml?identifier=3026060.

Chapter 2

Hahn WC. Role of telomeres and telomerase in the pathogenesis of human cancer. *J Clin Oncol* 2003; 21:2034.

Wright J, and JW Shay. Telomere biology in aging and cancer. *Am Geriatr Soc* Sep 2005; 53(9 Suppl):S292–4.

Bavinck JN, et al. Relation between smoking and skin cancer. *Am Soc Clin Oncol* 2001; 19(1): 231–8.

Bergfeld WF, and RB Odom. New perspectives on acne. *Clinician* 1996; 12:4.

Chapter 4

Smith R, N Mann, A Braue, G Varigos. The effect of a low glycemic load, high protein diet on hormonal markers of acne. *Asia Pac J Clin Nutr* 2005; 14 (Suppl):S43.

Van Leeuwen R, S Boekhoom, JR Vingerling, et al. Dietary intake of antioxidants and risk of age-related macular degeneration. *JAMA* Dec 28, 2005; 294(24):3101–7.

McNaughton SA, GC Marks, and AC Green. Role of dietary factors in the development of basal cell cancer and squamous cell cancer of the skin. *Cancer Epidemiol Biomarkers Prev* Jul 2005; 14(7): 1596–607.

Fitzpatrick TB, RA Johnson, K Wolf (eds), et al. *Color atlas and synopsis of clinical dermatology*, 3rd edition. New York: McGraw-Hill, 1997, 442.

Graat M, EG Schouten, and FJ Kok. Effect of daily vitamin E and multivitamin-mineral supplementation on acute respiratory tract infections in elderly persons: A randomized controlled trial. *JAMA* 2002; 288:715.

Wu X, GR Beecher, JM Holden, DB Haytowitz, SE Gebhardt, and RL Prior. Lipophilic and hydrophilic antioxidant capacities of common foods in the United States. *J Agric Food Chem* Jun 16, 2004; 52(12):4026–37.

Macheix J, A Fleuriet, and J Billot. *Fruit phenolics*. Boca Raton, FL: CRC Press, 1990.

Lazze MC, R Pizzala, M Savio, et al. Anthocyanins protect against DNA damage induced by tert-butyl-hydroperoxide in rat smooth muscle and hepatoma cells. *Mutat Res* 2003; 535(1):103–15.

Bagchi D, CK Sen, M Bagchi, and M Atalay. Anti-angiogenic, antioxidant, and anti-carcinogenic properties of a novel anthocyanin-rich berry extract formula. *Biochemistry (Mosc)* 2004; 69(1): 75–80.

Hou DX. Potential mechanisms of cancer chemoprevention by anthocyanins. *Curr Mol Med* 2003; 3(2):149–59. Review.

Roy S, S Khanna, HM Alessio, et al. Anti-angiogenic property of edible berries. *Free Radic Res* 2002; 36(9):1023–31.

Uehara M, H Sugiura, and K Sakurai. A trial of oolong tea in the management of recalcitrant atopic dermatitis. *Arch Dermatol* Jan 2001; 137(1):42–3.

Camouse MM, KK Hanneman, EP Conrad, and ED Baron. Protective effects of tea polyphenols and caffeine. *Expert Rev Anticancer Ther* Dec 2005; 5(6):1061–8.

Aneja R, PW Hake, TJ Burroughs, et al. Epigallocatechin, a green tea polyphenol, attenuates myocardial ischemia reperfusion injury in rats. *Mol Med* 2004; 10(1–6):55–62.

Mitscher LA, M Jung, D Shankel, et al. Chemoprotection: A review of the potential therapeutic antioxidant properties of green tea (Camellia sinensis) and certain of its constituents. *Med Res Rev* 1997; 17:327.

Sin BY, and HP Kim. Inhibition of collagenase by naturally occurring flavonoids. *Arch Pharm Res* Oct 2005; 28(10):1152–5.

American Academy of Family Physicians. AAFP Clinical recommendations. Available at: www.aafp.org/policy/camp/19.html.

Covington MB. Omega-3 fatty acids. *Am Fam Physician* 2004; 70: 133–40.

Nierenberg DW, RE Nordgren, MB Chang, et al. Delayed cerebellar disease and death after accidental exposure to dimethylmercury. *N Engl J Med* 1998; 338:1672.

Mercury levels in young children and childbearing-aged women — United States, 1999–2002. *MMWR Weekly* Nov 5, 2004; 53(43): 1018–20.

What you need to know about mercury in fish and shellfish. U.S. Department of Health and Human Services and U.S. Environmental Protection Agency, March 2004; http://www.cfsan.fda. gov/~dms/admehg3.html.

Summary of dioxins, furans, and PCBs in farmed salmon, wild salmon, farmed trout, and fish oil capsules. Food Safety of Ireland, March 2002; http://www.fsai.ie/surveillance/food/surveillance_food_summarydioxins. asp.

Glynn A, S Atuma, M Aune, PO Darnerud, and S Cnattingius. Polychlorinated biphenyl congeners as markers of toxic equivalents of polychlorinated biphenyls, dibenzo-p-dioxins and dibenzofurans in breast milk. *Environ Res* 2001; Section A 86: 217–28.

SCF (Scientific Committee on Food) (2001). Opinion of the SCF on the risk assessment of dioxins and dioxin-like PCBs in food — update based on new scientific information available since the adoption of the SCF opinion of 22nd November 2000 (CS/ CNTM/DIOXIN/20 REV 6 final).

Jacobson JL, and SW Jacobson. Intellectual impairment in children exposed to polychlorinated biphenyls in utero. *N Engl J Med* 1996; 335:783.

Research needed to reduce scientific uncertainty about effects of hormonally active agents in the environment. National Academy of Sciences, August 3, 1999; http://www.foodsafetynetwork.ca/pesticides/endocrine-disruptors. htm.

Rignell-Hydbom A, L Rylander, A Giwercman, et al. Exposure to PCBs and p,p'-DDE and human sperm chromatin integrity. *Environ Health Perspect* Feb 2005; 113(2):175–9.

Jacobs MN, A Covaci, and P Schepens. Investigation of selected persistent organic pollutants in farmed Atlantic salmon (Salmo salar), salmon aquaculture feed, and fish oil components of the feed. *Environ Sci Technol* Jul 1, 2002; 36(13):2797–805.

Hites RA, JA Foran, DO Carpenter, et al. Global assessment of organic contaminants in farmed salmon. *Science* Jan 9, 2004; 303(5655):226–9.

Brown DJ, and AM Dattner. Phytotherapeutic approaches to common dermatologic conditions. *Arch Dermatol* 1998; 134:1401–4.

Weber KS, KD Setchell, DM Stocco, et al. Dietary soy-phytoestrogens decrease testosterone levels and prostate weight without altering LH, prostate 5alpha-reductase or testicular steroidogenic acute regulatory peptide levels in adult male Sprague-Dawley Rats. *J Endocrinol* 2001; 170:591.

Sonee M, T Sum, C Wang, and SK Mukherjee. The soy isoflavone, genistein, protects human cortical neuronal cells from oxidative stress. *Neurotoxicology* Sep 2004; 25(5):885–91.

Kumar NB, A Cantor, K Allen, et al. The specific role of isoflavones in reducing prostate cancer risk. *Prostate* 2004; 59(2):141–7.

Li Y, KL Ellis, A Ali, et al. Apoptosis-inducing effect of chemotherapeutic agents is potentiated by soy isoflavone genistein, a natural inhibitor of NF-kappaB in BxPC-3 pancreatic cancer cell line. *Pancreas* May 2004; 28(4):e90–5.

Wei H, R Saladi, Y Lu, et al. Isoflavone genistein: Photoprotection and clinical implications in dermatology. *J Nutr* Nov 2003; 133(11 Suppl):3811S–19S.

Sudel KM, K Venzke, H Mielke, U Breitenbach, C Mundt, et al. Novel aspects of intrinsic and extrinsic aging of human skin: Beneficial effects of soy extract. *Photochem Photobiol* May–Jun 2005; 81(3):581–7.

Chan LY, PY Chiu, and TK Lau. An in-vitro study of ginsenoside Rb1-induced teratogenicity using a whole rat embryo culture model. *Hum Reprod* 2003; 18:2166.

Harmon, NW. Equisetum arvense. *Pharm J* 1992; 399:413.

U.S. Preventive Services Task Force. *Guide to clinical preventive services,* 2nd ed. Baltimore: Williams Wilkins, 1996.

Chapter 5

Nelson ME, MA Fiatarone, CM Morganti, et al. Effects of high-intensity strength training on multiple risk factors of osteoporotic fractures. *JAMA* 1994; 272:1909.

Suzuki K, et al. Systemic inflammatory response to exhaustive exercise. Cytokine kinetics. *Exerc Immunol Rev* 2002; 8:6–48. Review.

Feldman SR, et al. Ultraviolet exposure is a reinforcing stimulus in frequent indoor tanners. *J Am Acad Dermatol* 2005; 53:1038–44.

Chapter 6

Altemus M, B Rao, F Dhabha, et al. Stress-induced changes in skin barrier function in healthy women. *J Inves Dermatol* 2001; 117: 309–17.

Cohen-Zion M, and S Ancoli-Israel. Sleep disorders. In: Hazzard WR, JP Blass, JB Halter, et al. *Principles of geriatric medicine and gerontology.* 5th ed. New York: McGraw-Hill, 2003, 1531–41.

IMS Health. AC Neilsen survey, 2005.

The National Sleep Foundation is a national not-for-profit organization headquartered in Washington, DC, http://www.sleepfoundation.org/about/index.php?secid=&id=269.

National Institutes of Health State-of-the-Science conference statement: Management of menopause-related symptoms. *Ann Intern Med* Jun 21, 2005; 142(12 pt 1):1003–13. E-pub May 27, 2005. Review.

Hirshkowitz, M, CA Moore, CR Hamilton, et al. Polysomnography of adults and elderly: Sleep architecture, respiration and leg movements. *J Clin Neurophysiol* 1992; 9:56.

National Sleep Foundation. Sleep in America Poll. Washington, DC, 2002.

Rechtschaffen A, BM Bergmann, CA Everson, CA Kushida, and MA Gilliland. Sleep deprivation in the rat: X. integration and discussion of the findings. *Sleep* Feb 1989; 12(1):68–87.

Brown R, G Pang, AJ Husband, and MG King. Suppression of immunity to influenza virus infection in the respiratory tract following sleep disturbance. *Reg Immunol* 1989; 2:321.

Vgontzas AN, E Zoumakis, EO Bixler, et al. Adverse effects of modest sleep restriction on sleepiness, performance, and inflammatory cytokines. *J Clin Endocrinol Metab* 2004; 89:2119.

Spiegel K, E Tasali, P Penev, and E Van Cauter. Brief communication: Sleep curtailment in healthy young men is associated with decreased leptin levels, elevated ghrelin levels, and increased hunger and appetite. *Ann Intern Med* 2004; 141:846.

Gangwisch JE, D Malaspina, B Boden-Albala, and SB Heymsfield. Inadequate sleep as a risk factor for obesity: Analyses of the NHANES I. *Sleep* Oct 1, 2005; 28(10):1289–96.

Sarifakioglu N, A Terzioglu, L Ates, and G Aslan. A new phenomenon: "Sleep lines" on the face. *Scand J Plast Reconstr Surg Hand Surg* 2004; 38(4):244–7.

Kripke DF, NR Simons, L Garfinkel, and EC Hammond. Short and long sleep and sleeping pills: Is increased mortality associated? *Arch Gen Psychiatry* 1979; 36:103.

Grandner MA, and DF Kripke. Self-reported sleep complaints with long and short sleep: A nationally representative sample. *Psychosom Med* Mar–Apr 2004; 66(2):239–41.

Diagnostic Classification Steering Committee. *The international classification of sleep disorders, revised: Diagnostic and coding manual.* Rochester, MN: American Sleep Disorders Association, 1997.

Benca R. Mood disorders. In: Kryger MH, T Roth, and W Dement (eds). *Principles and practice of sleep medicine,* vol 85. Philadelphia, PA: W. B. Saunders, 1994, 899.

Vakkuri O, A Kivelä, J Leppäluoto, et al. Decrease in melatonin precedes follicle-stimulating hormone increase during perimenopause. *Eur J Endocrinol* 1996; 135: 188.

Schernhammer ES, CH Kroenke, F Laden, and SE Hankinson. Night work and risk of breast cancer. *Epidemiol* Jan 2006; 17(1):108–11.

Krauchi K, C Cajochen, and A Wirz-Justice. Thermophysiologic aspects of the three-process model of sleepiness regulation. *Clin Sports Med* Apr 2005; 24(2):287–300, ix.

Hernandez-Reif M, T Field, J Krasnegor, and H Theakston. Lower back pain is reduced and range of motion increased after massage therapy. *International J Neuroscience* 2001; 106(3–4): 131–45.

Chapter 7

Luecken L, E Suarez, and C Kuhn. Stress in employed women: Impact of marital status and children at home on neurohormone output and home strain. *Psychosom Med* Jul–Aug 1997; 59(4):352–9.

Parker J, SL Klein, MK McClintock, F Tausk, et al. Chronic stress accelerates ultraviolet-induced cutaneous carcinogenesis. *J Am Acad Dermatol* 2004; 51:919–22.

Chiu A, S Chon, and A Kimball. The response of skin disease to stress: Changes in the severity of acne vulgaris as affected by examination stress. *Arch Dermatol* 2003; 139:897–900.

Fawzy F. A short-term psychoeducational intervention for patients newly diagnosed with cancer. *Support Care Cancer* Jul 1995; 3(4):235–8.

Gura ST. Yoga for stress reduction and injury prevention at work. *Work* 2002; 19(1):3–7.

Chapter 9

Christenson L, T Borrowman, C Vachon, M Tollefson, C Otley, et al. Incidence of basal cell and squamous cell carcinomas in a population younger than 40 years. *JAMA* 2005; 294:681–90

Berman BM, L Lao, P Langenberg, WL Lee, AMK Gilpin, and MC Hochberg. Effectiveness of acupuncture as adjunctive therapy in osteoarthritis of the knee: A randomized, controlled trial. *Ann Intern Med* 2004; 141(12):901–10.

Chen CJ, and HS Yu. Acupuncture, electrostimulation, and reflex therapy in dermatology. *Dermatol Ther* 2003; 16(2):87–92. Review.

Andersson S, and T Lundeberg. Acupuncture — from empiricism to science: Functional background to acupuncture effects in pain and disease. *Med Hypotheses* 1995; 45:271.

Stern RM, MD Jokerst, ER Muth, and C Hollis. Acupressure relieves the symptoms of motion sickness and reduces abnormal gastric activity. *Altern Ther Health Med* 2001; 7:91.

Stephenson NL, SP Weinrich, AS Tavakoli. The effects of foot reflexology on anxiety and pain in patients with breast and lung cancer. *Oncol Nurs Forum* 2000; 27:67.

Bellometti, S, L Galzigna. Serum levels of a prostaglandin and a leukotriene after thermal mud pack therapy. *J Investig Med* 1998; 46:140.

Chapter 10

Bergfeld WF, RB Odom. New perspectives on acne. *Clinician* 1996; 12:4.

Adebamowo CA, D Spiegelman, FW Danby, et al. High school dietary dairy intake and teenage acne. *J Am Acad Dermatol* 2005; 52:207.

Chiu A, SY Chon, and AB Kimball. The response of skin disease to stress: changes in the severity of acne vulgaris as affected by examination stress. *Arch Dermatol* 2003; 139:897.

Harper JC. An update on the pathogenesis and management of acne vulgaris. *J Am Acad Dermatol* Jul 2004; 51(1):S36–8.

Roihu T, and A Kariniemi. Demodex mites in acne rosacea. *J Cutan Pathol* Nov 1998; 25(10):550–2.

Bonnar E, P Eustace, and FC Powell. The demodex mite population in rosacea. *J Am Acad Dermatol* Mar 1993; 28(3):443–8.

Crawford GH, MT Pelle, and WD James. Rosacea: I. Etiology, pathogenesis, and subtype classification. *J Am Acad Dermatol* Sep 2004; 51(3):327–41; quiz 342–4.

Wilkin J, et al. Standard grading system for rosacea: Report of the National Rosacea Society Expert Committee on the classification and staging of rosacea. *J Am Acad Dermatol* 2004; 50(6):907–12.

Wong RC. Physiologic skin changes in pregnancy. In: Harahap M, and RC Wallach (eds). *Skin changes and diseases in pregnancy.* New York: Marcel Dekker, 1996, 37.

Rhodes AR, MA Weinstock, TB Fitzpatrick, et al. Risk factors for cutaneous melanoma. *JAMA* 1987; 258:3146.

Weinstock, MA. Do sunscreens increase or decrease melanoma risk: An epidemiologic evaluation. *J Investig Dermatol Symp Proc* 1999; 4:97.

Index

Authors' Note

Sexy, Ageless Skin <u>Can</u> Be Yours!

**Visit www.beyondbotox.com
and go Beyond Botox
with these valuable interactive resources:**

- **Complimentary Samples & Advice:** Register at www.beyondbotox.com to become a Beyond Botox member and you will receive B. Kamins, Chemist, product samples and skin care advice targeted to *your* specific skin needs.

- **Beyond Botox 7-Step Program Worksheet:** Keep track of your lifestyle changes with the easy-to-use Beyond Botox 7-Step Program Worksheet. Download your copy at www.beyondbotox.com.

- **Q&A with Ben Kaminsky:** Get your answers from the chemist himself! E-mail your questions or concerns directly to Ben Kaminsky at info@beyondbotox.com. You will receive expert skin care advice from one of North America's preeminent dermatological chemists.

- **Fitness & Nutrition Resources:** Follow our helpful links to fitness and nutrition resources that will inspire your healthy lifestyle.

- **Success Stories:** Read testimonials from our seven-step program users or encourage others to go Beyond Botox by sharing your success story in our featured "Success Profiles."

How to contact us:

We'd love to hear from you with your questions, comments, and success stories about Beyond Botox and our seven-step program. Simply write to us at info@beyondbotox.com. We enjoy hearing your feedback and we promise we will read it.

Ben & Howard Kaminsky

To learn more about B. Kamins, Chemist, or their products, or to find a retail location near you, go to www.bkamins.com.

Hachette Book Group USA is not a sponsor of this offer and is not responsible for its content or the activities of www.beyond botox.com.

About the Authors

Ben Kaminsky, a preeminent pharmaceutical and dermatological chemist, has been developing medicines for physicians and dermatologists all across North America for over thirty years. Kaminsky continues to develop breakthrough formulas in the field of progressive skin care at Montreal-based Odan Laboratories, which he founded in 1974.

In 1997, Ben and his son Howard, a recent graduate of Notre Dame Law School, founded B. Kamins, Chemist, which has quickly become one of the leading skin care companies in the growing field of cosmeceuticals — skin care that bridges the gap between the dermatologist's and plastic surgeon's office and those products found at traditional cosmetics counters.

B. Kamins, Chemist, offers a unique and comprehensive range of products formulated for women and men of all ages. The product line includes a complete array of cleansers, toners, moisturizers, body care, masks, and reparative treatments.

Ben Kaminsky was the first chemist to specifically address the special skin needs of perimenopausal and menopausal women. The creation of the B. Kamins, Chemist, Menopause Cream and Menopause Body Lotion marked the first products of this kind specifically targeted to hormone-deprived skin. Kaminsky originally formulated the product for his wife and, after seeing the difference it made to the appearance of her skin, realized that many hormone-deprived-skin symptoms could be treated without prescription medicines.

Kaminsky is also a pioneer in treating rosacea, an acne-like inflammation that occurs in adults and manifests itself in red patches on the face. This condition, for which there is virtually no topical treatment, challenged Kaminsky to create B. Kamins, Chemist, Booster Blue Rosacea Treatment, a breakthrough therapy to help doctors treat rosacea when traditional products have failed.

Ben Kaminsky is a graduate of the Faculté de Pharmacie de l'Université de Montréal. He is an accomplished oil painter and takes great pleasure in caring for his award-winning gardens at his home in Montreal.

Howard Kaminsky, cofounder and CEO of B. Kamins, Chemist, oversees all aspects of domestic and international business, from sales and marketing to manufacturing and public relations. Kaminsky has over twenty years of industry experience encompassing senior leadership positions in practicing law, sales, operations, and product development.

Kaminsky partnered with his father, Ben (a leading chemist), to develop breakthrough formulas that focus on a range of skin conditions, with emphasis on sensitive, menopausal, rosacea, acneic, problematic, and extradry skin types. Before cofounding the company in 1997, Kaminsky held private law practices in both Montreal and New York City, serving such prestigious clients as Coach leather goods, Movado, and Laura Ashley.

Howard and Ben Kaminsky started B. Kamins, Chemist, by going door-to-door to different spas and locations in the Northeast and shipping products back and forth on Greyhound buses. Today B. Kamins, Chemist, a multimillion-dollar corporation, is located in six countries, with offices in Montreal and New York City and reps serving both the United States and Canada.